"*Eating the Moment* is a quick... ative, clever exercises and insigh... Rather than being shamed into d... original exercises to help them l... manage their appetites. Who kne... ~~...ght control could~~ be so fun and empowering?"

—Dina Cheney, author of *Tasting Club*

"In *Eating the Moment*, Somov gives you the practical tools you need to reap the rewards of eating more mindfully. Read it and discover how to have a relationship with food that is smarter, healthier, more conscious, and enjoyable."

—Deborah Kesten, MPH, author of
The Enlightened Diet

"Somov is one of the most creative psychologists around. He is knowledgeable about research-based and effective therapy techniques. He is aware of Eastern philosophies, and Buddhism in particular. And he is a productive therapist who knows how to translate knowledge into personal action for clients. All of these gifts are evident in Somov's book, *Eating the Moment*, which is not only informative, not only good reading, but also tremendously helpful in the most difficult area of behavior change—losing and keeping off weight."

—Stanton Peele, Ph.D., JD, author of
Seven Tools to Beat Addiction and
Addiction-Proof Your Child

"*Eating the Moment* is a thoughtful feast for those who want to understand the psychology of eating and how to overcome mindlessness with food. The 141 eating practices are easy-to-grasp appetizers for becoming more aware, overcoming craving, and transforming your experience with food. If you have ever wanted a primer on eating skills that you never learned at home or in school, this book is an excellent place to start.

—Donald Altman, author of *Meal by Meal* and *Art of the Inner Meal*

eating the moment

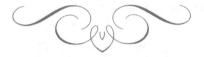

141
mindful practices
to overcome overeating
one meal at a time

PAVEL G. SOMOV, PH.D.

New Harbinger Publications, Inc.

Publisher's Note

Distributed in Canada by Raincoast Books

Copyright © 2008 by Pavel G. Somov
New Harbinger Publications, Inc.
5674 Shattuck Avenue
Oakland, CA 94609
www.newharbinger.com

Cover and text design by Amy Shoup; Acquired by Melissa Kirk; Edited by Brady Kahn

Library of Congress Cataloging-in-Publication Data

Somov, Pavel G.
  Eating the moment : 141 mindful practices to overcome overeating one meal at a time / Pavel G. Somov.
     p. cm.
  Includes bibliographical references.
  ISBN-13: 978-1-57224-543-3 (pbk. : alk. paper)
  ISBN-10: 1-57224-543-3 (pbk. : alk. paper) 1. Compulsive eating. 2.
Mindfulness-based cognitive therapy. 3. Food habits. I. Title.
  RC552.C65S63 2008
  616.85'260651--dc22

                          2008029817

14   13   12

10   9   8   7   6   5

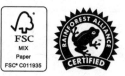

Contents

Acknowledgments

Just as the sun keeps on rising, books keep on being written and published. And so has this one, but not without help. I owe much gratitude to acquisitions editor Melissa Kirk, both for the discerning art of obtaining and for seemingly bottomless patience in chaperoning a novice author through the fjords of publishing. I owe gratitude to copy editor Brady Kahn for untiring tact and for oh-so-validating willingness to explore the original meaning of the author's choice of words. I owe gratitude to art director Amy Shoup for so precisely illustrating the satisfying intimacy of mindfulness with the cover picture that is, indeed, worth a thousand words. On a personal side of this "publishing matter," I owe gratitude to all who have nurtured my nature and to the countless "rascal sages" that I have encountered in life who have taught me lessons I did not seek to learn but—in retrospect—could not have afforded to go without. Thank you, all!

Introduction

Eating is complex. Overeating is even more complex. Both are problems. We have learned to solve the problem of eating with food. And we have learned to solve the problem of overeating with dieting. This book is about unlearning the solutions to overeating that have become problematic in their own right and about learning to start a habit of mindful eating. This book is for overeaters and overdieters.

The Mindful-Not-Mouthful Approach Isn't a Diet but a Diet Facilitator

The mindful eating (or, as I like to call it, the "mindful-not-mouthful") approach is an awareness-building and habit-modifying process for overcoming overeating; it is not a diet, at least not in the modern sense of the word. However, the approach can be used as a diet facilitator. Before I explain what I mean by the term *diet facilitator*, let me clarify what was originally meant by the word "diet." *Dieta*, in Latin, means "a way of living." Therefore, in its original meaning, a diet pre-supposes a *permanent* change in the way (or style) of life that preserves a way (or style) of life worth living. Geneen Roth, an anti-dieting pioneer and author of several best-selling books, suggests that for a diet to work, it cannot feel like a diet (Roth and Lamott 1999). While mindful eating can facilitate diet compliance, it is, at its basis, a *dieta*—a lifestyle or a way of living; by definition, it does not interfere with quality of life.

Most modern weight-management systems, known as "diets," are not quite diets in this sense. These diets can be subdivided into two distinct components or phases: an *induction phase* and a *maintenance phase*. The induction phase is a blitzkrieg of nonliving that usually involves some kind of drastic restriction of foods and portion sizes. If endured, the induction phase results in a relatively rapid weight loss. The maintenance phase is a recommended way of living that allows the dieter to maintain the target weight following the induction-phase weight reduction. With this distinction in mind, it could be said that the induction phase is not really a diet in the original sense of the word. Indeed, it would be hard to imagine anyone realistically maintaining an ascetic self-denying crash-diet regimen indefinitely and still call it "living." The maintenance phase, with its long-term focus and more realistic degree of self-restriction, is closer to the original meaning of the word "diet." The maintenance phase is not, however, what a typical overeater has in mind when he or she goes on a diet.

Most overeaters view dieting as the only solution and typically see it as a time-limited sprint toward weight loss, not a lifelong marathon toward health. As you go on a diet, you think tactically, not strategically: you are thinking not of a lifelong commitment to a particular way of living but, rather, of mobilizing just enough motivation and self-discipline to endure a sprint of self-denial so that you can fit into a reference-point piece of clothing, such as a pair of jeans worn in high school or a wedding dress or that spring-break bikini from sophomore year of college. Again, the mindful-not-mouthful approach is not a diet, but it can be used as a diet facilitator; it is an approach to living. The mindful-not-mouthful approach can be useful in facilitating both the induction and the maintenance phases of weight-management systems and other programs for overcoming overeating. As a diet facilitator, mindful eating is a resource you can cultivate before you embark on another diet (should there be a need for another diet in your future).

What to Expect and What Not to Expect

As an overeater, you may have wondered, what do people who overcome their overeating problems have that you lack? Willpower? I don't think so. Mindful, conscious eating, like any habit, has a learning curve and therefore is predicated on either trial and error or guided preparation. Some former overeaters learned their lessons through dieting, in which each diet became a learning experience, with its mishaps and revelations. Other former overeaters have sought professional help or read self-help books on overeating. Sooner or later, one way or another, people who overcome overeating develop a kind of personal eating know-how that consists of mindfulness and compliance strategies that allow them to adhere to their eating goals. The intent of the mindful-not-mouthful approach is to spare you the odyssey of trial and error.

In showing you these experiential shortcuts into mindful eating, I make the following promises. I will not ask you to count calories or to cut out any particular foods or to add any particular foods or to eat less or to eat more often or to exercise. Instead, I will be corruptly permissive. I will ask you to indulge yourself with new tastes and flavors. I will ask you to do strange but fun eating exercises. I will ask you to play and frolic with your food and your mind. Remember, you've got the rest of your life to overcome this problem! Kick back and find comfort in the notion that the success of the mindful-not-mouthful approach does not rest on willpower and self-discipline but on the profoundly human ability to reflect on your own experience as it progresses, that is, on the capacity for mindfulness.

Should You Use This Book If You Are on a Diet?

You know the cycle. Off another miracle diet for a few weeks, you have been "bad." Whether or not you lost weight while on the diet, you are intoxicated with the regained quality of life and freedom to eat whatever and whenever. But the high of this freedom has worn off as your guilt and aesthetic aspirations have started to poison the idyllic picture. A friend in the induction phase of her diet tells you about the pounds and inches she lost in just two or three weeks and suggests a book on the subject. Unbalanced or empowered by someone else's commitment and success, you venture out to your local bookstore. You browse around and stumble upon the title in question. You pick up the book, flip through it, and decide to buy it. This time, you're really going to do it. You pause for a moment, thinking about all the other diet books and exercise videos you've bought over the years, but then, just as before, you rationalize the expense of the book as an investment in your health. At home, you sit down to read it and then binge on one last feast before the self-imposed famine. After all, in just a few days, you'll be "good" again and sticking to the plan. Finally, pushing away from the table, you set a start date for the next diet, and off you go on another vicious round of self-denial.

Let it be different this time, dear reader: set no start date and make no promises. You're on a break, on a vacation from your previous diet, and on a contemplative retreat before your next diet, if, in fact, there is one. As part of my psychology practice, I periodically perform preoperative psychological evaluations for gastric-bypass surgery candidates. These clients' accounts of how they lost and regained hundreds of pounds of weight over the years have confirmed for me a long-standing clinical and personal realization: one of the main reasons why diets typically do not work is because they are sudden and impulsive undertakings. There's no gradual change. There is no practice, just the application. We jump into the role of a dieter after reading the script only once, without rehearsing our stage lines. We go from nondieting to dieting, from out-of-control eating to overcontrolled eating, expecting to have the best performance of our lifetime and the standing ovation of envious onlookers at the end. So, if you plan to go on another diet in the future, consider the mindful-not-mouthful approach as a kind of experiential boot camp.

Three Reasons Why We Eat

"Why do I eat?" This question—not the questions, "How much should I eat?" or "What should I eat?" or "When should I eat?" —is the logical starting point for anyone who is interested in overcoming his or her overeating. As I pose this question, you may take offense to the seemingly rhetorical nature of this inquiry. "Well," you might say, "I eat because I get hungry, to provide my body with energy." Congratulations, my fellow eater, and condolences at the same time! Congratulations for knowing the obvious and condolences for not living by the obvious. Yes, the grand biological idea behind eating is to pump fuel into our bodies to perform the functions of life. That is the theory! In practice, however, our reasons for eating often have nothing to do with the needs of our bodies. There are three reasons why we eat.

We Eat to Satisfy the Needs of the Body

We eat out of *physiological hunger*, a straightforward, undeniable need for fuel that results in *physiologically triggered eating*, the sole purpose of which is to satisfy the needs of the body.

We Eat to Satisfy the Needs of the Mind

We eat out of *psychological hunger*. Our minds need to be entertained, comforted, or distracted, resulting in *psychologically triggered eating*, the sole purpose of which is to satisfy the needs of the mind, even if the needs of the mind are satisfied at a cost to the body.

We Eat out of Habit

We eat without hunger, out of habit, when we are triggered to eat by various environmental stimuli that have been repeatedly linked with the act of eating. This mindlessly initiated, reactive, *environmentally triggered eating* mostly satisfies the insatiable food industry.

Four Reasons Why We Overeat

Voracious appetites and metabolic and lifestyle differences aside, on a behavioral level, overeating is maintained by the following four aspects of mindless eating:

- Mindlessness of the environmental triggers of eating

- Mindlessness of the process of eating

- Mindlessness of the sensations of fullness

- Mindlessness of emotional eating

Mindlessness Makes Sense but Not in the Case of Eating

On the surface of things, you might think that mindfulness is healthy and mindlessness is not. But if you look behind the curtains, into the complex mechanics of human function, into the multitasking miracle of human life, you realize that mindlessness makes sense. We are self-programming biological robots (with or without a soul, depending on our philosophical-spiritual orientation). To spare our minds the constant trouble of deciding on a myriad of trivial choices, to conserve energy, and to optimize performance, we automate ourselves. Eating is one such aspect of our functioning that we have automated. The problem with automated, and thus mindless, eating, however, is that conserving energy in today's sedentary world leads to obesity.

So as we focus on mindful eating, let us wave a fond farewell to mindless eating. After all, it is this mindless eating that helped us through many a business lunch where fully automated eating algorithms allowed us to skillfully handle pasta with red sauce only a foot away from the expensive tie of a prospective boss while rattling off bulleted versions of our work lives. It is this mindless eating that allowed us to have many a dinner date where we eloquently navigated through the courses of our relationship history without so much as a wine stain on our evening wear. It is this mindless eating that has allowed our blindfolded fingertips to find the last cashew in a jar of mixed nuts without so much as pausing the movie scene of a blindfolded man chewing through the ropes that

9

bind his hands. Let's face it: it's time to wave good-bye to mindless eating. We've had a good long run with it, a run that unfortunately slowed to a walk, then to a crawl, and finally to a limp on overburdened, aching ankles as we gingerly tread the mill of the weight-management track.

Mindful, Not Mouthful: Developing the Mindful-Eating Habit

The mindful-not-mouthful approach is designed to override the old habit of "if eating, then be mindless" with a new, more adaptive habit of "if eating, then be mindful." In a manner of speaking, the mindful-not-mouthful approach aims to automate mindfulness. Automate mindfulness? Isn't that a contradiction in terms? Not really. While the goal of making mindful eating a habit may seem paradoxical, it really isn't. The purpose of this book is to help you become habitually mindful of your eating, to get to the point where the decision to be mindful about eating is evoked mindlessly, automatically, effortlessly. Yes, I'd like for mindful eating to have the force of habit in your eating life. This kind of habit-forming or conditioning is how the book in your hands can help you make a lasting difference in your battle with overeating.

The Aspects of Mindful Eating

For most of us, eating is a mindless, unconscious, reactive, compulsive, automatic, mechanical, thoughtless, habitual, hand-to-mouth activity. We are, in a manner of speaking, eating zombies. The overarching goal of the mindful-not-mouthful approach is to awaken and reprogram eating zombies with new habits of paying attention to external (or environmental) factors that trigger them to start and stop eating, to internal (physiological and psychological), factors that trigger them to start or stop eating, and to their processes of eating. Put differently, the habit of mindful eating involves the following:

- Habitual mindfulness of environmentally triggered eating

- Habitual mindfulness of hunger and fullness

- Habitual mindfulness of the process of eating

- Habitual mindfulness of emotionally triggered eating

- Mindful (rather than mindless) emotional eating

You'll learn more about what all of this means in the chapters following.

From Knowledge of Mindfulness to Practice of Mindfulness

Mindfulness and knowledge are different things. Knowledge is informational awareness. Mindfulness is experiential awareness. To know something is different from experiencing the same thing. In your self-help readings or treatment encounters, you may have come across the advice to eat mindfully or "slow down your eating and be conscious of taste." Receiving this advice leads to informational awareness. Applying this advice creates experiential awareness.

I remember learning to do a backflip as a kid. First, I gathered information from my more acrobatic friends. Struggling for words and relying primarily on gestures and body language, they shared their know-how with me. Armed with this information, I tried doing a backflip and hurt myself a few times before I got it right. In retrospect, I realize that the information I gathered had essentially no value; as I tried to do a backflip, I was following no one's blueprint but enacting a kind of intuitive kinesthetic visualization that I had in my mind long before I consulted my friends. Having materialized that kinesthetic vision, I had acquired experiential awareness of how a backflip is done, my own know-how of the backflip that cannot be adequately expressed in words.

Knowing that you need to be conscious of your eating, or even trying a few times according to someone's prototype of mindful eating, is insufficient to change your eating habits. And yet, informational awareness is a vital precursor of change. Without having the comfort of knowledge about how to do a backflip, I would have probably never attempted it. It was only when I thought I knew how to do it that I felt the confidence to try it, which opened the door to the series of trials and errors that eventually led me to successfully land on my feet. The intent of this book is to help you make the three-point journey from *knowledge* to *practice* to the destination of *habitual application* of mindful eating; the goal is to permanently awaken the overeating zombie.

No, It's Not the First Book on Mindful Eating

Don't get me wrong. The idea that mindless eating is one of the mechanisms of overeating is not original to this author. Various self-help authors have offered the advice to eat mindfully. With rare exception, however, the coverage of mindful eating has been mostly focused on becoming more mindful of the process of eating, typically in the form of such common-sense advice as slowing down and taking time to savor your food. The mindful-not-mouthful approach uses mindfulness to manage overeating from a more panoramic angle and offers 141 awareness-building and habit-modifying exercises to provide an experiential journey into the essence of mindful eating. As such, this book goes a step beyond the regurgitation of classic Buddhist mindful-eating meditations.

How to Use This Book

This book is a combination workbook and textbook. It's both hands-on and *mind-on*. You'll notice icons next to the exercises. The awareness-building exercises highlight opportunities for mindfulness. Habit-modifying exercises allow you to modify your eating habits. Some of the awareness-building exercises also may be used to modify your habits. You can use this book in one of two ways. You can either follow the organization of the book, moving from theoretical rationale to exercises, or, if you wish, skip the salad course of theory and plunge right into the main dish of the exercises. The specific sequence of the chapters follows a certain logic designed to maximize your absorption of the material. With this said, however, feel free to roam through the book at random, as long as you expose yourself to most of the material. As with a circle, it does not really matter which way you go (left or right) as long as you go all the way around.

Three Levels of Reading, Three Levels of Benefit

In reading this book, you may benefit at the following three levels:

Knowledge level. If you merely read this book without engaging in any of the exercises, you will develop a better understanding of the role of mindfulness in overcoming overeating and successfully managing your weight. You will likely become less self-critical of your overeating and might develop insight into the problems with past diet-maintenance phases. You stand a modest chance of using mindfulness to reduce overeating or to increase regimen compliance in future weight-management attempts.

Awareness-building level. If you not only read this book but also engage in awareness-building exercises in mindful eating, you will have a better prognosis for reducing overeating in the long term. Furthermore, if you are on a diet while reading this book, you may use the awareness-building exercises as a kind of hand brake to help you stay on your diet.

Habit-modifying level. If you read this book and engage in both awareness-building and habit-modifying exercises, you stand to make the most progress in overcoming overeating. You may lose some weight while experimenting with the exercises, whether or not you are on a diet. Furthermore, you will also develop a personalized philosophy of eating that will serve to prevent relapses into overeating as well as guide your choice of the next diet, should you feel the need for one in the future.

A Note to the Skeptic

What type of reader will you be? How much effort do you think you will invest? To a large degree, that depends on your level of skepticism. With this in mind, let me make the following point. From one skeptic to another: be skeptical of your own skepticism! I know just what you're thinking: here we go again, another behavioral banality. Do not rush to foreclose on the potential utility of this book. What gives? You've been struggling with overeating for a while, so chances are you'll soon get on another diet. Before you do that, why not work on developing a habit of mindful eating that just might help you get more out of your diet, should you go on one? If you already are on a diet, then again, why not see if this mindful-eating stuff can help you get the most out of your current diet regimen? If you are in counseling, seeing a therapist (best contingency of all!), working on your overeating, you can share this book with your therapist as a resource for behavioral homework. And, finally, if your skeptical hesitation is driven by a concern for the New Agey East-meets-West implication of the title, please be assured that this book will not have you swallow koans and haikus for breakfast, but it will have you chew on a generous helping of practical ideas and behaviors.

CHAPTER 1

But Everyone Else Was Eating!

*Becoming Mindful of
Environmental Triggers of Eating*

To review, people eat for three reasons: to satisfy the needs of the body, to satisfy the needs of the mind, and out of habit. But what's a habit? Any habit can be understood as a stimulus-response relationship in which a stimulus is an element of the environment that triggers us to respond in a previously conditioned, mindless manner. For example, since movie theaters traditionally sell popcorn and soda, we associate going to the movies (stimulus) with eating popcorn and nursing a giant soda (response). When we eat out of habit in response to an external trigger, our eating is initiated upon the demand of the environment. The environment demands that we eat now. And we mindlessly oblige. When we let the environment decide when we should eat, we are, in a sense, surrendering the sovereignty of our conscious choice over eating as well as our common sense. It takes the mindlessness of habit to justify paying six or seven bucks for a cup of ice cubes and a handful of popped corn kernels when we aren't even hungry!

Eating Out of Habit Means Overeating

I owe it to you to make the following point painfully clear: Unless you are eating to satisfy the needs of your body, you are overeating. In other words, if you are eating out of habit, not out of hunger, you are eating more than you need. Wasn't so bad, was it? On to the next truism.

Environmental Triggers Initiate and Maintain Overeating

Say a friend invites you out to eat. You aren't actually hungry but decide to go along. Once at the restaurant, the sights and smells provoke an intense appetite. "I am famished!" you proclaim, unaware of the hidden evolution of a want into a need. The dinner is over and you feel full, but your friend isn't finished. She wants to look at the dessert menu. Minutes later, seduced by the pictures of decadent desserts, your appetite is kick-started and you're plowing through a monster slice of Death-by-Chocolate. What happened? You saw something appetizing and developed a desire for it, a craving so strong that it had the conviction of hunger. Sound familiar? The point is that the environment (a combination of people, places, and foods) can both trigger us to eat when we are not hungry (initial overeating) and maintain our eating past the point of fullness (continued overeating).

Why Did You Eat Just Now?

 We eat to satisfy the needs of the body, to satisfy the needs of the mind, and out of habit when triggered by environmental cues. In the week to come, explore your motives behind each eating episode. After you eat, ask yourself, why did I just eat? Was I actually hungry, or was I just triggered to eat by something in the environment? Did I eat to cope, to address my emotional needs? Keep track of the reasons behind your eating episodes. Write them down in a notebook. For example, if you ate out of hunger, note that your eating was "need based." If you ate to deal with stress, note that you "ate to cope." If you ate on a craving, after being triggered by an environmental cue, note that your eating was "environmentally triggered." If several different reasons coincide, try to determine the primary motive for eating.

Why Are You About to Eat Right Now?

 Before you eat, ask yourself the following questions: "Why am I about to eat? Am I actually hungry, or am I about to eat because I've been triggered by something in my environment? Am I about to eat as a way of coping?" After you clarify to yourself why you are about to eat, do the following: Eat. Or don't eat. Recognize that right now you have an opportunity to make a conscious choice. At this point, that's enough. Continue with this exercise for a week or for as long as it appears valuable to you.

Hunger vs. Craving: What's the Difference?

A craving is a pseudo-hunger signal that mimics hunger. Cravings prompt us to eat as if we were hungry when we actually aren't. Hunger is a physiological need with a physiological signature, a state of body. Craving is a want, a psychological state, essentially a thought of desire, a motion of the mind. Hunger is generic: you need food, any food that'll make hunger go away. Cravings are specific: you want a particular food. Tribole and Resch (1996) have aptly called cravings "taste hunger" (88). Hunger depends on your physiology. Cravings depend on the situational context. For example, if you weren't hungry but, after passing a fast-food place, suddenly developed a desire to eat, the chances are that this was a craving and not a state of hunger. Your body probably didn't change in the time that it took for you to drive past a fast-food billboard, but your mind easily could have. The exercises below will help you practice how to distinguish between hunger and cravings.

Hunger Essay

awareness
Write an essay about true hunger. It's possible that you haven't had the experience of true hunger for quite some time, if ever. If so, you'll need to do some research by letting yourself have this experience. Don't worry; once you feel true hunger, you can relieve it by eating. After consulting your physician about whether it's safe for you to delay a meal to experience a state of hunger, plan a day (preferably a day off) when you'll allow yourself to abstain from eating until you get hungry. Push the envelope a bit: allow yourself to get hungrier than you have in a long time. Once you're at a point

of rather intense hunger, first describe the experience in an essay, and only then, eat. Note the physiological signature of this moment of hunger (if any), reminisce about the last time you felt this hungry, and meditate on what this moment of hunger brings to your mind (emotionally, philosophically, spiritually).

Craving Essay

awareness Practice distinguishing between a state of hunger and a craving. In the days to come, when you feel like eating, read over your hunger essay and ask yourself, "Is this experience I am having right now a state of hunger?" If the experience doesn't feel like hunger and seems to be a craving, then describe it in an essay. Note what triggered your craving, what you are craving, and the duration of the craving (if it has already subsided). Will you satisfy your craving? Make a conscious choice: eat or don't eat. Note in your essay that you made a conscious choice to eat or not eat, but resist the temptation to specify which particular choice you made. After all, the idea is not to track your abstinence resolve but to help you differentiate your cravings from hunger and to practice making conscious choices about eating.

What Do You Crave Most Often and Why?

awareness What do you crave most often and why? Track your cravings to identify your craving patterns. To make sense of your craving patterns, ask yourself when, where, and under what circumstances you crave this. Do your cravings reflect a particular *exposure pattern* (such as craving a cappuccino when passing a coffee shop), or do your cravings correlate with a particular mood? My own craving for soup, for example, tends to vary with the illumination of a room: if the place is dim, I am prone to order soup. I jokingly call this a "seasonal affective appetite" (meaning that low lighting is reminiscent of cloudy winter days and affects the mood of my appetite). Enjoy this exercise as a treasure hunt into the patterns of your cravings. What will you do about the cravings? Practice the habit of making a mindful choice of whether to eat or not eat. At this point, making a conscious choice about eating is more important than the actual choice you make.

Craving-Driven Eating vs. Hunger-Driven Eating

Craving-driven eating may be conscious or unconscious. You might see food and eat it just because it's there, without even realizing it, which would be a case of mindless grazing. Or you might see the food, experience a craving, recognize that you are not hungry, and make a conscious choice to eat anyway. In contrast, hunger-driven eating is always conscious: hunger, as a physiological imperative, commands the presence of the mind.

Craving-Driven Eating vs. Hunger-Driven Eating

awareness Contrast and compare craving-driven eating with hunger-driven eating. Schedule a craving-driven eating day, where you eat each and every time you have a craving. On a separate hunger-driven eating day, eat only if you are hungry. On the craving-driven eating day, notice the process of social and environmental *synchronization*. When you eat in a craving-driven fashion, you eat each and every time the environment presents you with a powerful enough stimulus to elicit a craving in you. As a result, you become attuned to the environment, eating in sync, as if line dancing with a crowd of strangers. Everybody eats, and you eat. Compare this with a different kind of synchronization, *self-synchronization* (synchronization with yourself), when you eat in a hunger-driven manner. While you begin to feel progressively out of sync with the environment (everybody eats, but you don't), you start to get a sense that your behavior is becoming synchronized with your intentions. Notice which feels better to you.

Eight Common Environmental Triggers of Eating

All eating triggers (or the environmental stimuli that pull the strings of our appetite and provoke cravings) can be divided into the following eight categories: food characteristics, activities, settings (places), events, time, people, words, and weather. What are your eating triggers?

Trigger Detective

awareness

Follow the tracks of your foraging and grazing to find the environmental culprit of your craving. For the next two weeks, after you eat, ask yourself why you ate. If you ate out of hunger, you have nothing further to do. If, however, you ate out of a craving, then ask yourself what type of trigger it was that prompted your eating. After two weeks, draw conclusions about your key trigger vulnerabilities; for future reference, keep a record of your conclusions in a notebook. To remember your insights, think of a way to label your craving pattern. Are you a "stress eater," a "TV-watching eater," an "eater-outer," a "by-the-clock eater?" To help you better identify which trigger caused your craving, refer to the summary of triggers below:

Food characteristics: smells, sights, sounds

Activities: TV, reading, entertainment, thinking, problem solving, socializing

Settings: indoors (eating in, eating out), outdoors (backyard barbecue, picnic, drive-in)

Events: holidays, birthdays, weddings, parties, grief anniversaries, stress days, days off

Time: breakfast time, brunch time, lunchtime, dinnertime, suppertime, nighttime

People: permission people (foodie friends, parents, comfort/support people), stress people

Words: health words, taste words, food words, food-processing words (roasted, grilled), brand names

Weather: inclement weather, picnic weather

Food Characteristics That Trigger Eating

Some food characteristics, such as smell and taste, naturally trigger our appetite. Others, such as the look of food, may have an acquired craving-inducing power. Take the classic M&M's chocolate candy: with their waxy, artificial coloring, M&M's seem more like toys than food. Clearly, you first have to learn that these little multicolored marbles are food before you can actually crave them. Explore the trigger value of certain food characteristics and discover the sensory modalities that tend to activate your cravings.

Acquired Taste?

awareness Some food properties are innate triggers of eating while others are acquired through learning, exposure, and socialization. Let's try to tease out which ones are which. The method is simple: when you encounter a given food, ask yourself if you would have eaten it as a child. As a child, how do you think you would have responded to specialty cheeses, caviar, meat cooked rare, or coffee? As you do this hypothetical taste-testing with a child's palate, ponder the following question: if we can acquire a taste for something that we did not initially like, that is, if we can learn to turn a "yuck" into a "yum," can we also learn to turn a "yum" back into a "yuck"?

What Kind of Craver Are You?

awareness What sensory modality triggers cravings for you the most? Do you crave with your eyes or with your nose? Are you a *visual* or an *olfactory* craver? Or are you possibly an *auditory* craver, for whom hearing a description of a dish triggers more of a craving than seeing or smelling the actual food? Auditory cravers are really just visual cravers in disguise. Upon hearing a description of a food, the auditory cravers visualize it in the mind and crave this imaginary picture of it. Then, there are *tactile* cravers, who crave the touch, the texture, of food in their mouths. Since it's hard to crave pure texture independent of a particular food, tactile cravings are secondary to visual or olfactory cravings. First, you see a tub of yogurt and then you crave its smooth, light texture. First, you hear a description of a chocolate cake, and then you begin to crave the melting texture of chocolate. First, you smell a pizza, and then you imagine the stringy, chewy texture of cheese.

To test what kind of craver you are, get a handful of menus and a highlighter. After looking at the pictures in a given menu, highlight the words that have particular trigger power for you; then move on to the next menu. When done, analyze the results. What got to you more, the pictures or the descriptions? What were the sensory themes? Did you highlight the words that pertain to the look or the smell of food? If looking at the pictures in the menus and reading the descriptions of dishes didn't trigger any cravings, then you might be an olfactory craver; you might have to actually smell food to have your appetite triggered. Similarly, if you tend to lose your appetite when you have a cold and your nose is stopped up, chances are you are an olfactory craver. How is this useful to know? Depending on your craving sensory modality, your trigger avoidance strategy might be either "out of sight, out of mind, out of mouth," "out of nose, out of mind, out of mouth," or "out of earshot, out of mind, out of mouth."

Trick Your Nose

habit change If you have established that your preferred craving sensory modality is smell, try to throw off your sense of smell by applying a tiny bit of Tiger Balm or Vicks VapoRub to the tip of your nose. Track the results. Draw your conclusions. If the strategy works, use it as a habit-modifying or, to be exact, sense-modifying tool.

If you are an olfactory craver (if your nose plays a bigger role in your appetite than your eyes), then it might seem that you are at a disadvantage. Since you can smell food even if you don't see it, it is much harder to avoid the smell of food than it is to avoid the sight of food. Therefore, in addition to the "out of nose, out of mind, out of mouth" avoidance strategy, you might also have to reprogram some of your eating habits. For example, instead of the old "if it smells good, then eat it" idea, perhaps you could practice the new idea that "if it smells good, then smell it," and take your time to enjoy the smell. The fact of the matter is that smell does not have to be a trigger liability for you; if smell is your thing, then you might have to practice making a conscious choice to *just smell* rather than let smell trigger an eating response.

The Nose Knows

awareness To practice making a conscious use of your nose, consider keeping a diary of daily food smells that you come across. Allow yourself to practice fine-tuning your sense of smell so that you can actually use your nose to enhance the mindfulness of your eating process. By doing so, you will reprogram yourself to go beyond the knee-jerk "this smells good, therefore I want to eat it" response. Instead, allow your nose to imagine the kitchen from which a given smell emanates, let your nose explore the smell, and make educated guesses about the given foodstuff that you are smelling and the specifics and subtleties of its preparation. In short, allow your nose, triggered by a smell, to trigger you into a state of mindful savoring of the aroma. After all, smell is free. Enjoy the romance with the aroma, the special kind of chemistry that only your nose knows.

Activities That Trigger Eating

Many activities can trigger eating. The discussion below may help you identify the type of activities that trigger your appetite.

TV VIEWING

Watching TV and snacking is an entertainment formula that has thwarted many a diet. If, one day, TV manufacturers discover a way to make television emit smell (which they'll surely market as a "full-immersion experience" along with surround sound), our stomachs will start to resemble the boxy TVs of yesteryear.

To TV or Not to TV?

awareness To explore the trigger potential of TV viewing, compare two kinds of evenings—with TV and without TV. Don't worry: I am not asking you to eliminate TV altogether. On day 1 (TV day), first eat dinner and then watch TV for an hour. Note any cravings. On day 2 (the TV-free day), eat a meal comparable to the meal you had on day 1, and then have a TV-free hour. Note if you have any cravings during this TV-free hour and compare the number of cravings (if any) and their intensity with the cravings you had (if any) while watching TV on day 1. Also note whether and how much you ended up eating in the hour immediately after your meal on both days. For a meaningful comparison, this exercise will have to take place on two separate but otherwise similar days (weekday to weekday, stress day to stress day, weekend day to weekend day). So, to TV or not to TV? That is indeed the question of the times!

READING

Eating has come to augment our entertainment reading and to console us when we have to read as a chore, such as when studying or reading for work. Reading and eating has also enjoyed a cultural stamp of approval: a newspaper for breakfast symbolizes an idyllic morning. Even coffee houses, historically marketed as conversation forums, have become dull reading rooms where coffee no longer stimulates conversation but only accompanies you and your laptop.

No-Food-in-the-Library Rule

awareness &
habit change

Remember those "No Food or Drink" signs in the library and all the ingenious ways you tried to sneak in a sandwich or a candy bar? Here's a chance for you to be your own watchful librarian. The idea is simple: for a week, if you are in a habit of reading and eating, abstain from eating during reading and just read. In particular, copy this page, fold it to make a makeshift bookmark, and use it with the book you are currently reading. Bookmark your mindfulness with a mindfulness bookmark. Read to feed your mind, not your mouth. Let reading create food for thought rather than thoughts about food. Try this out for a day or two. If you find this to be a meaningful exercise, try food-free reading for a week.

ENTERTAINMENT

Traveling circuses, gladiator fights, and theatrical performances of the past may have made way for today's sporting events, rodeos, dog/horse/car races, and moviegoing, but the combination of the visual and the gustatory remains the same. While the times have changed the menus, the marriage of entertainment and food appears to be everlasting.

SOCIALIZING

Family dinners, dinners out with friends, business lunches, diplomatic receptions, neighborhood barbecues, and romantic picnics are some of the classic forms of social eating. Sure, eating is a good way to bond; after all, hunger is a common denominator. But for some families, couples, and groups of friends, eating has become a relational crutch. Don't get me wrong: I don't mean to suggest that you become a hermit and never share a meal with anyone. Just beware of the danger of the collective appetite. And consider cultivating noneating common denominators in your relationships.

Peer-Pressure Eating

*awareness &
habit change* Are you a social eater? Do you tend to eat when others eat? Do you primarily socialize through eating out? Do you

try to please people by agreeing to their invitation to eat when you are actually not hungry? Do you tend to overeat when you eat in company? Monitor your social-eating habits for a couple of weeks to gauge the impact of company on your appetite. If you feel you are easily susceptible to peer pressure to indulge, rehearse some assertive yet tactful limit setting. Tip: if overeating during work lunches has been a particular issue for you, try eating lunch solo and, to maintain the relationships, offer instead to go for a walk with your former lunch partners.

THINKING AND PROBLEM SOLVING

When you have something on your mind, it's not unusual to end up with something in your mouth. Problem solving, as a work-related activity, often leads to eating. Somebody calls for a brainstorming session, and before you know it, the think tank becomes the eat tank. Do we think better when we eat? Or do we just defend against the chore of thinking by the comfort of eating? Ponder and monitor this under-recognized trigger of overeating in the weeks to come.

Places That Trigger Eating

Have you noticed how eating in the kitchen can differ from eating in the living room, how eating in differs from eating out, how eating out at a backyard barbeque differs from eating out at a company picnic? Not only is our eating triggered by certain places, but also certain places trigger different rules of eating engagement, as well as the amounts we are socially sanctioned to eat.

A Study of Appetite Manipulation

awareness Eating establishments are professionally designed to stimulate your appetite for eating, whether you are hungry or not. Restaurants, cafes, bistros, bars, and diners are craving booby traps with the greatest convergence of eating triggers. Go to a nearby eating establishment to conduct a systematic study of appetite manipulation. Get something to eat (to avoid undue attention) and mentally catalogue the elements of the environment (from the décor to the menu) that you think are designed to manipulate your appetite. Conduct a few such field trips to identify the most craving-inducing landmine of an eating establishment. Decide if you wish to avoid it in the future. You can also think of an "eating establishment" as simply any place where you eat most often. Your own eating establishment may be anywhere in your home, a certain recliner, the kitchen, your bedroom, or your work desk. What place have you turned into an eating establishment by associating it with eating? Ponder this and draw conclusions.

Events That Trigger Eating

In addition to various calendar events (such as holidays and birthdays), days of the week can serve as mini-events that determine the way we eat. For years my own cravings for desserts seemed to vary by the day of the week. In trying to make sense of that pattern, I had to consider the psychology of dessert. From the physiological standpoint, dessert is an absolutely unnecessary dish. Psychologically, however, dessert is a form of indulgence, if not self-care, and thus serves to remind us of the sweetness of life. With this in mind, it is of little surprise that my craving for dessert would parallel my need for stress relief. Consequently, on Mondays, if I had a particularly daunting week ahead of me, I'd crave dessert as a way to offset the work dread. Similarly, on weekends, dessert made sense because that was when, I thought, we were supposed to rest and indulge ourselves. As my thoughts about work and weekends have changed over the years, so have the patterns of my cravings for dessert.

A Fiesta, Not a Feast

habit change Have you noticed that we tend to celebrate with food? Celebrations are a powerful, culturally sanctioned trigger to eat, overeat, and even binge-eat. For many overeaters, food-centered holidays are a dreaded challenge and a source of post-holiday rumination and self-dissatisfaction. Here's a new paradigm to try: have a fiesta without having a feast. The word "fiesta" originates from the word *festus*, which is Latin for "joyous." The essence of a holiday is celebration. Eating is but one way to celebrate. Try to experiment with celebrating a holiday in a way that is not food centered, in a manner that is joyous but not necessarily gluttonous. Pick a calendar holiday or a personal event, preferably something that is coming up soon, and make it a fiesta, not a feast. For example, instead of going out to eat to celebrate your birthday, have a picnic. Eat, commune with nature, throw a Frisbee. This way you'll have a celebration that will involve some eating but won't be primarily food focused. Start simple: if heavy eating has been a long-standing tradition at a particular event, such as a family reunion, then you may want to leave it as is, at least for now. You can practice this fiesta-not-feast mentality on a more personal occasion, where the format of the celebration is fundamentally your prerogative. Relational anniversaries and birthdays are perfect opportunities to experiment. Aim to develop a standing tradition of celebrating some calendar and personal events in a non-food-focused manner.

A Fast, Not a Feast

habit change Fasting as a means of celebrating is as old as the world. Much has been written about fasting, and I encourage you to develop some curiosity about it. For the purposes of this exercise, the term *fast* shall refer to a continuum of eating restrictions, ranging from complete food-free, water-only fasting to various dietary restrictions, as you would find, for example, in the tradition of Lent. Before undertaking this exercise, be sure to read up on the health benefits of fasting and consult your physician about whether fasting, to any degree, is safe for you. Select a calendar, personal, anniversary-based, or spiritual/religious holiday and commit to a fast (whatever would be appropriate for your level of health) prepare for it, and conduct it on the day in question. If you find fasting on a holiday to be a more meaningful experience than feasting, consider a yearly tradition of at least one fast-not-feast holiday.

Times of Day That Trigger Eating

Times of day also trigger our eating. When we eat almost never has anything to do with when we need to eat. We are socialized to refer to the time clock, not the body clock. We eat in the morning, not because we are hungry but because we are supposed to have breakfast in the morning. We lunch around noon, not because we necessarily need food at that time but because it is lunchtime and lunchtime, by definition, is for eating lunch. We arrange our suppers around family members' schedules or TV shows. Times of day not only trigger us to eat but also influence how much we eat, which is a physiologically absurd situation. Imagine filling up your car with gasoline because you consulted the clock instead of your gas gauge. You would simply decide it was time to pull into the gas station and fill up the car, regardless of whether the car has gone anywhere or stayed in the garage. Even more absurd, during a certain point of the day, you would fill it up with an extra amount of gas. Why? Just because it's that time of day! Of course, this approach would not work with cars, given their limited tanks. But, don't worry, our stomachs—our ever-expandable fuel tanks—can handle a little topping off!

The Times of Our Eating Lives

awareness

For a couple of weeks, keep track of when during the day or night you eat and whether when you eat, in fact, coincides with when you feel hungry. Also, track how much time you spend eating in any given day. For an additional insight, tabulate the overall amount of time (in months or years) that you have spent masticating over your lifetime. Also, consider experimenting, if only for a couple of weeks, with shifting from a time-based decision to eat ("it's time to eat") to a physiologically more intuitive idea ("I am hungry enough to eat now").

People Who Trigger Eating

Eating around some people is almost instinctive; around others, eating is a matter of coping. Some just exude a kind of permissive quality that allows us to relax, be ourselves, and not have to bother with self-monitoring. Others will offer you food until you are groggy because they don't know how else to connect with you or how to manage their own anxiety. And then you have these stressful people whose very presence triggers emotional eating. Explore who influences your eating habits and choices.

People Who Influence Your Eating

awareness   Ask yourself the following questions:

1. "Who triggers me to eat well? Who encourages me to eat mindfully, to savor, to eat healthy?"

2. "Who triggers me to indulge, overeat, or go off my diet or regimen? Who gives me the permission to be 'bad'? Who urges me to enjoy myself only to justify his or her own urge to binge?"

3. "Who triggers me to stress-eat, binge-eat, cope-eat, react-eat? Whose presence do I cope with by eating?"

4. "Who is my 'junk-food person'? Who always dials up for a pizza or taunts with french fries?"

5. "Who is my 'sweets person'? Who bakes cookies, invites me out for ice cream, or always brings in doughnuts?"

6. "Who in my life needs me to eat in order to connect with me? Who expresses his or her love for me through feeding me?"

7. "Whose eating do I influence?" List names.

Words That Trigger Eating

Words are powerful triggers: they compel us into action every day. What words trigger your eating? Explore these linguistic triggers and group them into the following categories: health words ("antioxidants," "high fiber"), diet words ("zero calorie," "no sugar," "low fat"), taste words ("creamy," "delicious," "rich"), food words ("chocolate," "ice cream"), food-processing words ("freshly baked," "freshly squeezed," "hand picked," "broiled," "roasted"), and brand words (brand words need no introduction). As an exercise, list the words that trigger your eating.

Weather as an Eating Trigger

There is something appetite provoking about inclement weather. Have you noticed a pattern of craving comfort food when it rains or snows or storms outside? Perhaps it's about a sense of control: by making ourselves comfortable inside, we defy the harshness of nature, persuading ourselves that we can survive it, that we can stay in control of life, despite nature's unpredictability. Explore whether weather influences your appetite and how.

The Toolbox: How to Control Cravings and Triggers

There are two broad approaches for dealing with environmentally triggered eating: *trigger control* and *craving-control*. Trigger control helps you avoid triggers that provoke your cravings as well as reduce their trigger power through a process of desensitization. Craving-control helps you manage the cravings once they arise. These two approaches are complementary: to get across the temptation landmines without blowing up (your waistline), you must learn to avoid the avoidable triggers and control the inevitable cravings. These two approaches consist of at least six separate strategies: two trigger-control strategies of *trigger avoidance* and *trigger desensitization* and four craving-control strategies of *distraction*, *self-talk*, *relaxation*, and *mindfulness*. We'll begin with craving-control strategies first. The reason is simple: since one of the trigger-control strategies involves purposeful exposure to triggers, you will need a good skill base in craving-control to help you avoid any unnecessary overeating. Before beginning, you need to take an inventory of your current craving-control strategies.

How Do You Control Cravings Now?

awareness Each day you encounter multiple eating triggers. How do you resist the temptation to eat when you are hungry? How about when you are not hungry? Do you have a craving-control method, or do you just wing it? Do you smoke to suppress your appetite? Do you use self-talk? Distractions? Or do you just white-knuckle it? Summarize your craving-control know-how. Analyze what works for you and what doesn't. Take a few minutes to learn from your craving-control successes. What successes? Look, chances are that in your life you've controlled more cravings than you haven't or, at least, far more than you think you have. Give yourself credit for the craving-control foundation that you've already put into place. And you can build on that!

The Four Strategies of Craving-Control

One of the most common and most intuitive craving-control strategies is distraction. The strategy of trying not to think about eating often backfires, however, since not thinking about something usually means thinking about it even more. Self-talk, another traditional craving-control strategy, involves the use of self-motivational statements that reiterate the benefits of sticking to a plan and remind you of your health goals. Self-talk, in its reliance on logic and reason, is of limited utility: craving is an emotional state that takes the otherwise rational brain and reduces it to irrational simplicity. Rational self-talk is hard to pull off when your mind's wisdom has been reduced to a nutritional tantrum of "I want!" Breath-based relaxation for craving-control is an improvement on either distraction or self-talk, as it allows the craving-aroused mind to return to its rational baseline. Mindfulness, as a craving-control technique, involves just witnessing or just noticing craving thoughts as they pass. Mindfulness has received much clinical attention, particularly in the area of substance-use treatment, where the goals of relapse prevention closely parallel the challenges faced by chronic overeaters (Marlatt 2002a).

Not All Craving-Control Strategies Are Created Equal

In my opinion, mindfulness and relaxation are the first echelons of craving-control, followed by self-talk and distraction strategies. But don't just take my word for it: experiment with all four to make an informed choice. If you decide to stick with self-talk or distraction, the exercises in this chapter will allow you to modify these strategies to leverage more craving-control value out of them.

Some Helpful Hints

There are many ways to combine the four craving-control skills. My favorite combinations are mindfulness plus relaxation and relaxation plus self-talk. Experiment with combining these skills and don't be afraid to get creative. Here are some other helpful hints.

TAKING THE GUESSWORK OUT OF CRAVING-CONTROL

You can try out the four different methods for controlling your cravings and track your impressions on their effectiveness. Doing so will help you take the guesswork out of craving-control. This way, instead of trying to improvise a craving-control strategy on the fly, in the future you will be able to use a craving-control method that you've tested and found to be effective.

TAKING THE EXPOSURE RISK

Any exposure to triggers creates an opportunity to practice your craving-control strategies. Purposeful exposure accelerates the learning curve. Therefore, two ways to expedite craving-control training are *imaginary exposure*, which involves imagining an eating-related trigger, and *in-vivo exposure*, which involves actively seeking out real-life eating-related stimuli.

Craving-Control Through Mindfulness

Mindfulness, as a craving-control method, involves two essential mechanisms: passive attention and dis-identification. What is *passive attention*? Attention can be either active or passive, that of an active observer or an uninvolved witness. Say, I lost my house keys. I would have to look for them. But in the process of looking for my house keys, I might also happen to see an old concert ticket. Mindfulness is about seeing, not looking for, something. It is about just noticing and just witnessing, without an attachment or identification with what is being noticed and witnessed. This latter element is called *dis-identification*.

When you identify with something else, you are relating, drawing a sign of equality between yourself and the other thing. When we experience a craving, there is a risk of getting lost in it, becoming overwhelmed. And yet cravings come and go. For us to identify with something that is inherently transient and fleeting is to lose our sense of self, a sense of our immutable continuity. This kind of identification with something impermanent is what imbues craving with suffering. Mindfulness allows us to recognize that a craving is but a part of the overall experience, a transient, fleeting state of mind, not the mind itself. Mindfulness practice teaches you to realize that this thought, this feeling, this sensation (whatever it might be at any given moment) is but an object inside your mind, no more significant than a paper cup on your kitchen counter. Yes, it is a part of you, but it's not all of you. A craving is no more a part of your mind than a reflection of your face is a part of the mirror. And that's exactly why you can just notice it, just see it, without having to stare at it. Mindfulness, as a craving-control method, takes less effort than the other methods. Unlike distraction, you are not pushing aside thoughts of food. You are letting go of any attempt to block them and, instead, are letting them in and just noticing them as thoughts and sensations. Unlike self-talk, you are not trying to change your mind but are accepting your mind as just mind. Unlike relaxation, you are not trying to calm yourself down from the excitation of the craving but are calmly accepting your excitation as just a part of the craving. In sum, mindfulness is a form of controlling by letting go of control.

The Mind Lava Lamp

awareness

You've probably seen a lava lamp. It's a sealed see-through container with a glob of wax submerged inside a liquid. As the liquid warms up from the power source, the wax melts and begins to float up and down, morphing into various shapes. The mind is like a lava lamp. Close your eyes right now for a moment and notice your thoughts, feelings, and sensations. All of this mind content is not unlike a glob of wax that moves and morphs from one form to another. Your awareness of this content is not unlike the liquid inside the lava lamp that surrounds the ever-changing glob of wax. And then there is you—the container of all these mental gymnastics. For this exercise, borrow or purchase a lava lamp. In the weeks to come, spend some time watching it. Turn on the lava lamp and just sit and watch. First, watch the glob of wax come to life. Notice it morph and change. Then, after a while, watch the liquid that surrounds the glob of wax. Watch it remain the same. Then, close your eyes and watch your *mind lava*—the thoughts, feelings, and sensations—the content of your mind. Allow yourself to think something like the following: "Wow, all these thoughts and feelings inside of me … and here's one … and another one," and so on. Then, after a while, become aware of your awareness of this mind lava. Allow yourself to have the realization: "Here I am, being aware of my thoughts and feelings coming and going. These thoughts and feelings are just like an ever-morphing glob of wax inside the liquid of my conscious awareness. And while these thoughts and feelings morph and pass, I—the I that is aware of all this internal commotion—remain the same." Rest assured that if you feel confused, you're actually on the right track. Just go ahead and watch the mind lava flow past you.

Counting Craving Thoughts

Next time you have a craving, pop into the nearest restaurant and order a cup of tea, but keep the menu. Bring a piece of paper and a pen with you. Look around, smell, look at the pictures in the menu, and watch your mind. Notice the craving thoughts, the food-related thoughts of desire, and each time you notice a craving thought, note it by making a dot on a piece of paper. Spend at least five minutes watching your mind like this while making dots on the paper, one after another. As you do this, you might compare your mind to a stream or a river and yourself to a dispassionate observer who is sitting on the bank of this river, watching the craving thoughts pass down the stream, staying put where you are, without getting carried away. As you watch these cravings come and leave, take note of your mindful presence in this moment: here you are, just noticing the craving thoughts, not going anywhere, staying in the moment, not fleeing, remaining fearless. Finish the exercise by counting the craving thoughts. Ponder the result: you have controlled all these craving thoughts by not controlling them, just by being nonreactively aware enough of them to allow them to pass. Congratulations! Practice this at home (staring at a food you like). Should you satisfy your cravings after you have mindfully managed them? That's really for you to decide.

It's Just a Craving, for Crying Out Loud!

awareness

If you feel that these mindfulness exercises are a bit too esoteric, here's a chance to get real. It's time to practice *mindfulness bravado*! Set yourself up to have a craving (I am sure you know how). As soon as you have a craving, first put on your calm mindfulness cap: notice the food; don't identify with it. Think, "This is just a craving. I am not a craving. This craving is just a part of me, a fleeting, transient, ephemeral, insignificant part of me, not even worth my attention." Then add a touch of mindfulness bravado: do not just notice, but notice with the kind of scorn that does justice to the insignificance of this mental event. After all, it's just another craving, one of thousands. And, indeed, where's the crisis? Where's the fire? You've been through this before; it's just the same old banal stimulus-response connection in your brain. You saw something, it triggered you to have a craving, and so here you are, having a craving thought. Feel the scoff, throw in some attitude: "A craving—whoop-de-do! So what if it lasts! Have I ever had a craving that didn't go away? Of course not! This too shall pass. Craving, my ass!"

Craving-Control Chair

habit change Habits (healthy or unhealthy) thrive on cues. To develop a habit of craving-control, I'd like for you to begin to work on creating a craving-control routine. Begin by choosing a location for craving-control in your home. This will be particularly useful for after-work or late-night cravings. More specifically, identify a particular chair in your home, a chair you will use for craving-control. That's really all there is to it. By designating a specific location for controlling cravings while at home, you are creating an environment of familiarity, an environment that will, with time, become associated with craving-control success. Having a place of this kind can help you build a tradition of confidence. With time, the craving-control chair will become a useful anchor to ground and center your craving-ridden mind. And, of course, avoid eating in the craving-control chair at all costs. Tip: for a long-term application of this sitting skill, I invite you to use the lotus or semi-lotus position as your craving-control chair. After all, when it comes to mindfulness, it's not about what you sit on or where you sit; it's that you sit. Let alone that the lotus chair is portable enough for all your life's moves.

Craving-Control Success Record

habit change Another step toward developing a habit of craving-control is to monitor your success. Get a pocket-sized notebook. Create a table of three columns. Label the first column "Date/Time" and the second column "Craving Intensity (0 to 10)." The third column is for writing down which particular craving-control strategy or combination thereof you used to control a given craving. You can use the first letters of the words "self-talk," "distraction," "relaxation," and "mindfulness" (such as "M+R" for a mindfulness/relaxation combination). Such a record will help you develop a sense of mastery and debunk the idea that you can't resist a craving. You will know through personal experience that you have repeatedly and reliably managed cravings of varying intensity. What constitutes a craving-control success? It is making a craving go away completely, even if only for a moment. Take pride in your success. Whether or not you eat after you have killed the craving is irrelevant. This is a diary of craving-control success, not a food log. Aim for a hundred craving kills. Periodically, review the mounting evidence of your craving-control prowess.

Mindfulness + Relaxation: A Master Skill for Craving-Control

habit change This exercise introduces you to my favorite craving-control combination, that of mindfulness plus relaxation. There are several ways to combine these two strategies: you can relax first and then use mindfulness for any residual craving thoughts, you can use mindfulness first and then relax, or you can use mindfulness and relaxation more or less at the same time. I call this the "dots and spaces" method. To try this method, begin by triggering a craving. Think about some food you like or, better yet, expose yourself to it directly, in-vivo. Then get a piece of paper and a pen, and put on your mindfulness cap. Notice as craving thoughts arise: each and every time you notice a craving thought, make a dot on the piece of paper. Do this for a few minutes. Then take a look at your drawing: it's a series of dots and a series of spaces. Each dot represents a craving thought that you registered on the radar of your awareness. Now, here's a question for you: what does the space between the dots on the paper represent? In other words, what were you thinking in between the craving thoughts that you had? Probably just other noncraving thoughts.

Now give this space (in between the craving thoughts) a different function. This time you won't need to mark anything down with a pen. Trigger yourself again with a food craving, sit down, close your eyes, and let your hands rest comfortably on your thighs. Begin to watch your mind for craving thoughts. When you notice the first craving thought, tap your index finger on your thigh (as if making a dot on a piece of paper) and immediately focus on the up-and-down movement of your chest as you inhale and exhale. Chances are that another craving thought will disrupt your breath-focus. If so, mindfully notice the thought and mark it by tapping your index finger on your thigh, and immediately refocus on the breath-space in between the craving thoughts. Do this until you have no more craving thoughts, until you comfortably rest in the breath-space of calm mind. Follow this approach for a couple of weeks.

Craving-Control Through Relaxation

A craving is a state of stress: you want something, but you're ambivalent about whether to have it or not. It takes effort to balance on the fence of indecision. Relaxation helps you get off the fence, down to the ground of certainty, back to your psychophysiological baseline.

Breath-Focused Relaxation

awareness & habit change
You may already be familiar with breath-focused relaxation. If so, you can skip ahead. If not, here are two no-nonsense,

easy-to-use relaxation techniques. The first is a breath-awareness exercise. Find a place to sit down, and close your eyes. Give yourself the permission to do nothing. After all, despite all the things you have on your plate, you have made the time to do this, so ... do this. Begin by watching your breath. Note the up-and-down movement of your chest, the in-and-out movement of your stomach, the fleeting breezy sensation of the air flowing in and out of your nose. Simply notice. Resist the temptation to manipulate your breath. Your lungs know how to breathe. Trust your body to find a slower and more restful pace of breathing. Just watch and observe. Let your breath pace deepen on its own. Feel free to shift from one type of breathing sensation to another. After a while, allow yourself to acknowledge that there are two opportunities for a pause: right after you inhale, before you exhale; and right after you exhale, before you inhale. Take the latter one: allow yourself a brief moment of rest after you exhale, right before you inhale. Don't force yourself to hold your breath. Just pause for a moment. As you exhale and your stomach sinks, merely settle into a momentary pause before you inhale again. That's it. Do this for a few minutes.

The second breath-focused relaxation exercise involves a degree of intentional breath control. Close your eyes and place one of your hands on your stomach. Notice how your hand moves up and down slightly as you inhale and exhale. Begin to take slightly deeper breaths, as if trying to move your hand a bit higher as you inhale more deeply. Take six to twelve such abdominal breaths. If you don't notice any relaxation, keep on going with more breaths until you do. That's it. Practice both exercises for a couple of weeks.

Exhale the Craving

habit change Having practiced the two previous breath-focused relaxations, try applying them to craving-control. There are two ways to proceed: trigger yourself to have a craving, or wait for a craving to arise in the natural course of your day-to-day living. In either case, use relaxation to control the cravings. More specifically, as the craving develops, take six to twelve abdominal breaths (or more, if necessary) until the craving is gone. You might find it useful to envision inhaling relaxation and exhaling the stress of the craving: in— relaxation; out—the craving. Alternatively, just focus on the sensations of your breath until your breathing begins to slow down on its own, and/or take advantage of the opportunity to pause after you exhale. If you are practicing at home, you can use your craving-control chair. Also, remember to document your progress in your craving-control success diary. Note relaxation as the method of choice while you practice this exercise, and if you'd like, keep track of how long it takes for you to breathe your way out of a craving for later cross-method comparisons.

Craving-Control Through Self-Talk

Self-talk is what you tell yourself, and it comes in two formats. *Inner dialogue* self-talk is an internal pros-and-cons analysis. When people use this strategy of self-talk to combat cravings, they often describe it as a polemic between a *pro-behavior voice* ("a devil on one shoulder") and an *anti-behavior voice* ("and an angel on the other shoulder"). These two voices engage in verbal combat as they duke it out over whether or not to engage in a given behavior. *Mental cheerleading* is a form of self-talk that consists of motivational catchphrases ("You can do it!") and self-coaching confidence-boosting statements that you repeat to yourself mantra-style.

Talk Yourself Out of a Craving

awareness &
habit change

Next time you experience a craving, try to talk yourself out of eating. List the pros and cons, mentally or in writing. Use your craving-control chair, if at home. Duke it out; see who wins. Note if self-talk actually reduces the craving intensity. In my experience, even when resulting in a decision not to eat, self-talk does not always reduce the intensity of the desire. Track what happens and document your progress in your craving-control success record.

Create a Self-Talk Script

habit change Self-talk, as a craving-control method, is usually improvised. But you can leverage the usefulness of self-talk by formalizing it into a script. Brainstorm various self-affirmations, self-motivational statements, catchphrases, health-oriented slogans, and wellness party lines ("Eat to live, not live to eat"). Combine the most poignant ideas into a self-talk script. Write them down and practice this self-talk script until you memorize it. Next time you have a craving, try to talk yourself out of eating by repeating to yourself your entire self-talk script, mantra-style. Document your progress.

Record and Play Back Your Self-Talk

habit change Record your self-talk script and get into a habit of playing it back both preventively, when you anticipate cravings will arise, and in response to cravings. Experiment with shorter and longer versions of the self-talk script. Take charge of programming your mind. Tip: if you are struggling with overeating at night, listen to the script on the drive home to get into a healthy state of mind as you walk through the door.

Craving-Control Through Distraction

To try to control your cravings, you can purposefully divert attention away from thoughts of food onto something else. As common as it is, distraction is highly underutilized. Three problems limit its craving-control power. The diversions are often not intense or involved enough to steal our attention away from thoughts of food. When attempted, they are often prematurely abandoned. And the diversions themselves often trigger cravings to eat, as would be the case if you decided to distract yourself from thinking about food by watching TV. Experiment with the following distraction-improvement exercises.

Distraction-Extraction Exercise

awareness

A successful craving-control diversion is a behavior that removes (extracts) you from the trigger zone and jolts (distracts) your mind into thinking about something entirely different. How does a cold shower sound to you? Too extreme? I doubt you've ever eaten in the shower or fantasized about food while there. And I bet that even ten seconds of cold water can reset your mind from craving a cookie to craving a warm towel. Where do you go from here? The challenge is to identify a distraction-extraction behavior that you can actually live with. You will need this for the following exercise. Search and you will find.

Craving Destruction Through Distraction

habit change If the cold shower idea was a bit extreme, I hope you found a suitable alternative. Let's field-test this diversion strategy. Trigger yourself to crave and use distraction to destroy the craving. Demolish and diminish it by taking an unambiguously vigorous course of action. Leave the scene of the craving; extract yourself from the trigger environment. Preoccupy yourself with something active and physical to distract your mind. And stick with it for at least fifteen minutes. No premature reentries into the trigger zones here if you want the distraction to work. If you decide to go cerebral and distract yourself from the craving by listening to music, crank it up and dance for at least three tracks; if you want to distract yourself with a crossword puzzle, yell out the words at the top of your lungs. Have fun and track your progress.

A Master-Skill Combo vs. a Combo Meal

awareness As a fail-safe, combine two craving-control skills to make one craving-control master skill. You can experiment with several different craving-control combos. I highly recommend the mindfulness/relaxation combo. Also try relaxation/self-talk, relaxation/distraction, and perhaps self-talk/distraction. Follow the same trial-and-error trigger-and-try method of exposure you've used so far. Think of this as the craving-control finals. Procure your forbidden fruit. Bring it home. Let it tempt you. Allow the craving to develop. Try out the different master-skill combos. For example: relax and then distract, or use your self-talk script and then relax, or try mindfulness and relaxation at the same time. Decide on what combination works best for you. Eat the trophy. Resume your life unafraid of cravings.

Developing a Craving-Control Habit

habit change Review your craving-control experiences: what craving-control methods or combinations did you like the best? Which method worked the fastest and felt most natural? Which method seems most socially portable and suitable for application in public? Whatever it might be for you, make a conscious commitment to use your chosen craving-control method as a craving-control default. Shopping for craving-control is over. Congratulations: you've taken the guesswork out of craving-control. Time to cultivate a craving-control habit. How? Through more practice, of course. The trigger desensitization exercises on the following pages will offer you plenty of opportunity to do just that.

Trigger Control: Trigger Avoidance and Desensitization

Trigger avoidance is simply staying away from the people, places, and things that trigger your appetite. "Out of sight, out of mind, out of mouth," I like to say, or, if you are an olfactory craver, "out of nose, out of mind, out of mouth." As difficult as it may be to create a drug-free environment, however, a food-free environment simply doesn't exist. Let's face it: food is the legal drug, and, as such, it is omnipresent. Despite its limited utility, however, trigger avoidance is not without some value, and some of the exercises that follow will allow you to tap this strategy for its maximum value. *Trigger desensitization* is a process of getting so used to a given trigger that it no longer has the power to trigger a craving. Repeated exposure to a particular trigger eventually rids it of its stimulus value. Eventually you stop noticing and reacting to the trigger. That's how you learn to tune out the midnight train whistles if you live next to a railroad track. An example of trigger desensitization would be to carry a bar of chocolate on you at all times. With this constant access to the object of your desire, you eventually learn to eat chocolate at your discretion, when you choose to eat it, rather than at random, whenever you encounter it in the environment.

Hungry Eyes

awareness This is an exposure exercise designed to help you desensitize yourself to your trigger foods. First, review the gustatory vulnerabilities that you discovered by doing the trigger detective exercise in this chapter. Then, get dressed, remove the money from your wallet (leave your buying power at home), and go to the nearest store that sells your trigger foods. While there, browse, endure, lose interest, leave. Practice walking away. If necessary, use your craving-control strategy of choice. Granted, unless you are willing to panhandle, you are really at no risk for acting on your cravings.

Hungry Ears

awareness This exposure exercise will help you desensitize yourself to the sound of food, or, to be exact, to the sound of people talking about food. Hearing others describe food can be a potent trigger. On Sundays, tune in to the NPR show *The Splendid Table*. Allow yourself to sit at this splendid table of gustatory delights and witness your cravings emerge. Listen, endure, and learn that cravings come and go, that you don't have to act upon your cravings, and that with time even the most splendid triggers lose their craving-inducing luster. If necessary, use your craving-control strategy of choice.

Food Shrine

awareness — *Flooding*, or an overwhelming degree of exposure, can expedite desensitization. To flood yourself with exposure, build a food shrine. As you do this, I encourage you to ponder how we worship certain foods. First, tell your significant others about this kooky exercise and get their informed consent. Then prepare your materials (pictures, articles, recipes of your favorite food, a personal poem about it). Then, build your shrine. If possible, place a sample of the actual food in the center of the shrine (take precautions to prevent infestation). Then, spend some time "worshipping" at the shrine on a daily basis. Allow the cravings to emerge. Let the exposure flood you. If necessary, use your craving-control strategy of choice. If, after a week, the experience continues to be meaningful, update the shrine with a new sample of food. Contemplate your insights.

You may repeat this exercise with another trigger food if you'd like.

Food Doesn't Have to Mean Eating

The meaning we assign to the objects around us predetermines their function: a tomato in the hand of a chef means food, whereas a tomato in the hand of a heckler means feedback. You see, the objects that we collectively refer to as "food" can mean other things besides being edible. Learning to recognize these other uses and meanings allows us to break the overconditioned associations between food and eating. Here are some ways to look at food as something other than food.

Food as art: inhaling life into nature morte. Food is both the subject of art and an artistic medium. Browse through your local art-life offerings in search of food as art. Check out the museum eateries that offer haute cuisine to art patrons hungry for a gustatory interface with the world of art. The idea here is to broaden your definition of enjoyment from gustatory to aesthetic. Whereas in the past, the only way you enjoyed food was by eating it, seeing the art in food will allow you to enjoy food without eating it. Also, experiment with the genre of still life (or *nature morte*). Pick a nice-looking apple and use it as a model for a drawing rather than an object to eat. Make a gingerbread skyscraper. Sculpt an elephant out of dough. Weave a braid from freshly made pasta. Carve a canoe from a baguette.

Whether your artwork will be in good taste or not, the point is to appreciate food as art without always having to taste it.

Food as function: the orange paperweight. Aside from nutritional and aesthetic value, food can also have a utilitarian function. Try using an orange as a paperweight and a warm tea bag as a compress on your temples or to blot your eyes. Slice up some cucumbers for a facial mask. Use a plastic-wrapped strip of beef jerky as a bookmark. Take a pair of square-shaped loaves of bread, allow them to get stale or stick them in the freezer; once hard, use them as push-up blocks for exercise. In short, creatively explore the nonnutritive utilities of food.

Food as product: the delicious profit margin. Whereas you eat to live, a food manufacturer lives off what you eat. Take a look at food as a commercial product: tour a farm or a food-processing plant; observe the dynamics of a pizza shop through a window. Consider the markups, the issues of distribution and storage. Consider how brand names offer us membership in a particular lifestyle or reflect certain values. Isn't it ironic that by surrendering to marketing, you, in effect, listen to the businessperson behind a food product as much as you would to your physician? After all, marketing is nothing other than a food manufacturer's attempt to influence your decision making about what you put into your body. In sum, look at the food through the eyes of a businessperson, and try to see how you, the consumer of food, fit into this picture.

Food as work: produce the produce. Food is work. If you haven't cooked, take up cooking. Try waiting tables or catering (for pay or on a volunteer basis). Grow a tomato. Wash dishes. Take a moment to ponder the chain of human effort that has produced the produce in your salad bowl.

Food as medicine: a spoonful of antioxidants. Food is medicine. We can treat ourselves to a cookie, or we can treat ourselves with a clove of garlic. What do you see when you see a serving of food? A portion or a dose? A disease or a cure? A poison or a medicine? Study foods' medicinal properties. Self-medicate; don't just eat.

The Carrot Cake Fight

awareness Get a carrot cake and a roll of paper towels. Drive out to a secluded area in the country. Pack a "snowball" out of a chunk of the moist carrot cake, aim at a tree, and throw. Notice how well the carrot cake packs into a ball. Repeat until the cake is gone. Yes, I have, indeed, lost my mind. Otherwise, why would I suggest something this bizarre, right? But hold your judgment: let's just say you went along with this; do you think you'd ever look at carrot cake again the same way? Of course not! Before this, carrot cake meant only one thing: "Eat me." Afterward, it will still mean "eat me," but it may also mean "throw me." The point is that food doesn't just have to mean eating. To expand on this exercise, come up with a creative way to interact with your favorite food so that stuffing your face with it is no longer the only fun option at your disposal. (A tip: if you find yourself licking the carrot cake off your hands, use your craving-control strategy of choice, or just use the paper towels.)

Trigger Avoidance: To Avoid or Not to Avoid?

awareness To avoid or not to avoid triggers? To answer this question, try for just one week to avoid as many of the identified triggers of your overeating as you can. You might have to change the route of your commute, avoid the break room at work, or stop watching TV. If you live with others, you might have to ask them to change some things as well. Perhaps, they'll agree not to buy certain types of foods or, at least, not to eat them in front of you. Who knows how you might have to rearrange your life and the lives of those around you to avoid exposure to all the things that trigger you to overeat?! Notice the growing confinement of your life's topography, all the people, places, and things you have to avoid. Can you eliminate some unnecessary exposure to triggers and, at the same time, avoid any downside or lost quality of life? Give this approach a systematic try and decide if it's a viable trigger-control strategy for you or whether it's a strategy to avoid.

People, Places, and Foods

habit change If trigger avoidance works for you, here's an opportunity for you to make enduring, habit-modifying changes. Review the trigger detective exercise and list the following information: the "permission" and "stress" people who trigger you to overeat, the places and settings that trigger you to overeat, and your trigger foods. Permanently reprogram your social routines (eliminate contact with your trigger people), your logistical routines (avoid those restaurants where you overindulge), and the topography of your daily living (change your commute route and where you spend time in or out of home). Trigger-proof your life by avoiding the avoidable exposure to your specific trigger trio of people, places, and foods.

No-TV Diet

awareness & habit change TV is a power trigger for overeating. Let's quantify the impact of television viewing on your eating patterns. There are three levels to this exercise. Level 1: Eliminate the TV from the menu, and go on a no-TV diet for a week.

For one week prior to eliminating TV, keep a diary of everything you eat. Then unplug your TV, or, better yet, put it in storage, and try the no-TV diet for a week. Write down everything you eat during this TV-free week. Level 2: Keep the TV, but cut out the programs that trigger you to overeat. Keep track of everything you eat during this week. Level 3: Keep the TV, but eliminate the TV commercials. Watch movies or commercial-free programming. Once again, keep a food diary during this commercial-free week. Compare the four food diaries. By now, you should have food diaries from a full TV-access week, a TV-free week, a trigger-programming-free week, and a commercial-free week. Draw your conclusions about the level of TV restriction you'd like to try on a long-term basis.

Need-Based Eating

habit change Whereas environmentally triggered eating is craving driven, need-based eating is hunger driven. To experiment with need-based eating, you'll have to define a couple of parameters. First, decide how many meals a day you wish to be driven by hunger (rather than your cravings). Say you decide to apply need-based eating to supper only. In that case, instead of just automatically planning on supper, you'd ask yourself: "Am I hungry? Do I actually need to eat right now?" If not hungry, then you'd skip supper. In this manner, you can choose to eat one or two meals, or, possibly, all of your meals on the basis of need. Next, decide how long to commit yourself to this experiment. You might decide to attempt need-based eating for one day, or you might decide to give it a week or a month. You could even decide to extend the time frame to an entire lifetime. Alternatively, you could decide that you will eat in a need-based manner during the workweek and not bother with need-based eating on the weekends (to balance health concerns with quality of life). At any rate, start off modestly. Note that the habit-modifying value of this exercise increases as you increase your degree of commitment (from one day to one week to one month to one year to one lifetime) and as you increase the comprehensiveness of your need-based eating (from one meal to all meals). Experiment; don't obsess. This is not a diet or a meal-restriction regimen but merely an opportunity for you to learn more about the need-based eating paradigm.

Regaining Control

The challenge is to awaken the eating zombie. The goal is ambitious but feasible: to help you break the behavioral chains enslaving your appetite to environmental cues and triggers and to regain control over when you eat. The aim is to help you shift from mindless, craving-driven, environmentally triggered eating to eating that is guided by conscious choice. Do you sometimes feel like a marionette, stuffing your face at the whim of an environmental puppet master? Can you eventually get back to just eating, no strings attached? Yes! After all, it's you, your mind, that has given the environment the power to pull the strings of your appetite! You can work on getting this power back.

CHAPTER 2

Becoming Mindful of the Process of Eating

A meal is an event; eating is a process. Whereas chapter 1 dealt with hunger as a point of departure, and chapter 3 deals with fullness as the destination, chapter 2 is about the experiential journey of eating and the sensory scenery between hunger and fullness. This chapter will focus on *how* we eat, on the experience of eating.

One-Track Minds

Activities such as watching TV or socializing both trigger eating and distract from it. The reason is that we can only consciously process one event at a time. True, it doesn't seem that way as we manage to breathe, engage in a three-way conversation over dinner, skillfully manipulate food, and tap our feet under the table, all at the same time! As the mind rapidly shifts attention from one activity to another, we experience the illusion of parallel engagement in several activities at once. Despite our mental agility, we are still disappointingly one-track. In a sense, the mind works like a flashlight: When you point a flashlight at an object in a dark room, that object emerges from the darkness, as if coming into existence. But when you move the flashlight away, the object—as far as your perception goes—ceases to exist. If you can't see it, it doesn't exist; if it doesn't exist, you can't experience it. When we eat and watch TV or talk, our minds are in a constant tug-of-war between the incoming stimuli competing for a chance at existence. In this ping-pong for attention, the mind loses conscious experience, and eating is reduced to a mindless hand-to-mouth behavior that we carry out with the unconsciousness of breathing: inhaling food by the mouthful.

Pragmatic Hedonists

Aside from the unflattering one-track nature of our minds, the ever-accelerating pace of our lives prompts us to become pragmatic hedonists. With little time to spare, we try to optimize each moment of leisure in order to amplify the total pleasure experience. It is no longer enough just to have something good to eat; we want a side of conversation with that. Unfortunately, this too leads to a loss of conscious experience. A delicious dessert is gone without enjoyment as our eyes are fixated on the tube, and a great TV moment is lost on us while we dip fries in ketchup.

When You Eat, Eat: Antidistraction Exercises

You might have heard the advice: when you eat, eat. But simply eating can be quite boring. That is, it can be, if you eat mindlessly. The following exercises explore the tedium of mindless eating to help you develop an appreciation for the stimulation of mindful eating.

Boring Eating

awareness Mindless eating is uneventful and, frankly, boring. The boredom of mindless eating is best illustrated by eating in the complete absence of distractions. Arrange to be alone, serve yourself a typical amount of food, close your eyes, and just eat. Note the emerging sense of boredom, the desire for stimulation. Avoid entertaining yourself mentally by rehashing the events of the day. Just eat. Imagine what it would be like if you had to eat like this all the time. Do you really think you'd struggle with overeating? Activities that fail to excite us do not result in behavioral excesses.

Eating Out Solo

awareness Go out to eat by yourself. In doing so, leave your newspaper behind, avoid the endless study of ketchup bottles or beverage menus, and, if you can, avoid the window seat to prevent street watching as a substitute for television. Try not to chat with the food server more than necessary. While there, just eat. Chances are you'll be out of the eating establishment in record time with a hefty take-home container. Draw your conclusions.

Distraction-Free Eating

awareness & habit change What's your most mindless and distraction-rich meal of the day? Family dinner with its cross talk? Or a bedtime snack with a TV remote in your hand? Or the work lunch spent surfing the Internet with a growing pile of bite-sized bags of Doritos and MoonPies from the vending machine? Identify your most distraction-laden meal of the day and try to endure it without any distractions at least once a week. As you do this, you might catch yourself thinking something absurd along the following lines: "Well, what's the point of eating right now if I can't watch TV?" Think of all the books that have been closed exactly at the moment when a reader's fingers found the last potato chip or the last M&M at the bottom of the bag! If interested in modifying your eating habits, aim to build up from one distraction-free meal per week to one distraction-free meal per day.

The Four Mindfulness Targets

In the process of eating, there are four mindfulness targets: the flavor, the movements of eating, the meal script, and the meal setting. Each of these four targets has a complexity of its own that warrants separate coverage. I'll begin with the aspect of flavor.

Mindfulness of Flavor: Taste, Smell, and Texture

Flavor is not the same as taste. In fact, it's an overall impression of the three different elements: taste, smell, and texture. Taste is communicated by four taste receptors on your tongue that detect sweetness, bitterness, sourness, and saltiness. Smell is communicated by olfactory sensors in your nasal passages and is thought to account for a significant portion of the overall experience of flavor. The texture, or feel, of food is also an important part of its flavor. To begin exploring flavor more fully, do the following taste-analysis exercise.

Recognizing the Four Aspects of Taste

awareness & habit change   When you sit down to eat your next meal, let the first order of your awareness-building business be to check for sweetness, bitterness, sourness, and saltiness. If you dare, taste-analyze a sample of different brands of dark chocolate. Don't panic; it's okay to eat chocolate; the only taboo in this approach is mindlessness. If your palate is anything like mine, you are likely to detect varying degrees of balance among sweetness, bitterness, and saltiness. What combination of these do you like the most in chocolate? Repeat this taste-test with different foods to train your palate. Pretend that whatever you are eating, you are eating it for the first time. Allow your tongue to become a tool of curiosity, a guide to sensation, rather than just a shoveling mechanism. As a habit-modifying exercise, consider routinely performing a taste-test whenever you eat something new. Or, for habit-modifying value, you could make it a point to recognize the four tastes—analyze for sweetness, saltiness, sourness, and bitterness—at the outset of each meal, with every dish you eat.

Chemesthesis: Texture

Chemesthesis is a phenomenon in which the food in the mouth, in addition to acting on the taste receptors, also acts upon the receptors for other senses, such as touch (Green, Alvarez-Reeves, and George 2005). Thus, the mouth conveys tactile information about the texture of the food, such as whether the food is solid, liquid, crumbly, creamy, or crackly, and whether it is drying, cooling, evaporating, irritating, spicy, or astringent in its mouth-feel. The sensory experience of food's flavor is a treasure trove of mindfulness opportunities.

The Subtext of Texture

 awareness & habit change

The texture of food can play more of a role than its actual taste. Chemically speaking, ice cream of a given flavor should taste the same, whether it is hard or soft, and yet it doesn't. To understand the subtle subtext of food texture, the mind needs categories. This is an opportunity to develop a vocabulary of texture so that you can begin to read its subtext as you eat. In the weeks to come, pause to assess the texture of what you are eating. What kind of mouth-feel does this food have? Watery, airy, creamy, tough, soft, crumbly, crunchy, silky, chewy, flaky, stringy, grainy, spongy, oily? If these words don't fit, and you find yourself in an obsessive tip-of-the-tongue search for the right description, that's great: after all, this is a struggle for mindfulness.

Expectation as an Element of Flavor

Our first sensory impression of a food often comes from its packaging. This is called *sensation transference*, a situation in which we project (transfer) our sensory experience of the product's package onto the product itself. In a classic example, Louis Cheskin, a marketing guru, increased the market acceptance of margarine by wrapping it in foil to suggest high quality (Gladwell 2007). This case of marketing hypnosis shows that our expectations about a food product are, in a way, an element of flavor.

Blind-Tasting

awareness As soon as we see food, we know what to expect tastewise. And as soon as we know what to expect, we stop paying attention. This makes sense: the mind is a kind of curmudgeon that doesn't like to waste its attention span on anything that it already knows. Unfortunately, this is how we shortchange our eating experience. While seeing is believing, seeing isn't always knowing. Take the seeing out of eating to bypass your preconceived notions about food and to rediscover the flavor of otherwise familiar foods. Have a friend bring an opaque container with a few food items inside. Put on a blindfold and allow your friend to feed you a bite of something. Note the increase in the mindfulness you bring to the table. Without seeing what you eat, you'll have to rely on the moment-by-moment awareness of the various components of the food's flavor, such as taste, smell, and texture. Take turns surprising each other. In the future, also consider consciously closing your eyes for a moment as you enjoy food. Make a note of how this kind of eye closing sometimes happens on its own, briefly, when we "mmm" in appreciation of a flavor. It seems that this curmudgeonly mind knows to close its eyes to savor, after all.

From Mindlessness to Recognition to Savoring

Tasting (or flavor recognition) and *savoring* are related but not the same. Savoring begins with tasting. Tasting is sensing. Savoring is enjoying what you are sensing. The following exercises will help you further develop your palate to enable you to mindfully enjoy your favorite foods. These exercises first serve to help you tune in to the flavor. And once tried for the purposes of flavor recognition, they can be used as vehicles for savoring.

Recognizing the Specific Ingredients

awareness & habit change

To become more mindful of taste, begin to identify and isolate the specific ingredients of food as you taste it. Remember that many foods and most dishes consist of multiple foodstuffs, and that each of the ingredients has its own gustatory signature. Try, for example, to distinguish between the taste of chocolate, ice cream, whipped cream, nuts, and the cherry as you work your way through a sundae. Go beyond the mere realization that you like the overall flavor to a degree of taste resolution that allows you to identify and evaluate the specific ingredients. "What's this that I'm tasting?" is the question to ask when eating something you have not prepared for yourself. Study the flavor: "Hmm, there is a nice sweetness to this sauce. I wonder if it's roasted pepper." For habit-modification value, carry a pocket notebook and use it to guess the ingredient list of a given recipe; whenever possible, match your guess against the menu description or information you obtain from your server. Treat this as a gustatory riddle to unravel or a friendly competition, if eating out in company. Make it fun: give yourself a code name ("Taste Cracker" or something goofy like that) and keep track of your progress.

Taste Essay

awareness

Select a food to sample, and then set out to systematically describe it—in writing. Start by describing the chemical taste: note whether the given foodstuff is sweet, sour, bitter, or salty, and in what proportion, and whether it is at all spicy. Describe the smell of the food as well. Then, describe the elements of the physical taste, such as texture and the temperature of the dish. Initially, jot down the words that describe the overall experience of the food and then integrate these descriptors into a taste narrative. You can turn this exercise into a Guess-the-Food parlor game. For example, you can read descriptions of three different types of berries to your friends and have them guess the berries on the basis of your descriptions. Following this, you can offer your friends the actual berries and walk them through the taste with a real-time narration of why such-and-such gustatory profile is an accurate taste essay for a given food substance.

The Essence of Flavor

awareness Arrange a plate with fresh strawberries, a piece of strawberry cake, a scoop of strawberry ice cream, and a piece of strawberry flavored chewing gum. Try a series of tastes to track down the strawberry factor. Ask yourself: What is the essence of strawberry? Is the strawberryness expressed in the smell, taste, texture, color, or temperature? Would I recognize the taste of strawberry in a piece of strawberry-flavored chewing gum if it came in green, not red? If strawberry isn't your thing, try to track down, say, the fish factor in fish dishes. What is the essence of the fish flavor? Asking these questions is more important than answering them. Chances are that the answers will remain mostly unverbalized, evading definition like a hundred-year-old catfish evading the hook. And that's okay. The point, after all, isn't whether your mind can catch the essence of a fish in a net of linguistic categories but that you endeavor on a fishing expedition into the mindfulness of flavor.

Assessing Your Taste Memory

awareness Gladwell (2007) describes the so-called triangle test of taste memory. An example of this test is the Pepsi Challenge. You present a subject with two plastic cups of cola, one containing Pepsi and another containing Coke. You have the person try to guess which is which. Say your subject has successfully passed the test. The triangle test is the same test but with a twist: you present someone with two glasses of one beverage and one of another beverage (for example, two glasses of Pepsi and one of Coke). The challenge is to identify the glass that has no double. Apparently, only a third of those tested are able to do so correctly (Gladwell 2007). What makes the triangle test a special challenge is that in order to succeed, you have to be able to somehow hold on to the taste impressions of the first and second glasses in your mind as you move from the first taste to the second and then on to the third.

This ability to hold on to a taste is *taste memory*, a specific application of sensory memory. To memorize a fading sensory experience, the mind has to be taught a process for breaking the overall taste impression into accessible categories. Professional food tasters develop "a vocabulary of taste," which allows them to understand and remember a taste for future comparisons (Gladwell 2007, 182). To assess your memory taste talents with the triangle test, you'll need plastic cups of three different colors. Have a friend pour two cups of one kind of beverage and one of a second beverage while he or she keeps track of which color corresponds to the mystery beverage (to the one that has no double). You could try this test with Pepsi and Coke or with two brands of comparable mineral water (perhaps Pellegrino and Perrier). Or you could do this test with two different brands of yogurt. To maximize your chance of success, mobilize your mindfulness: as you taste and sip, slow down, allow yourself to prolong the encounter with the flavor in order to understand and remember its essence.

Developing Taste Memory

awareness When we remember an event, we tend to see an image of that event in our mind. But what do we remember when we remember a taste? Usually nothing. Or just the fact that we liked the taste, which isn't the same as remembering the actual taste. While taste memory is typically the province of food-testing professionals, here you have a chance to practice "holding" a taste experience in your mind to try to cultivate this elusive skill. Try a tiny taste of whipped cream, meditate on its taste and mouth-feel, then spit it out and rinse your mouth. Close your eyes and try to recall the experience. Let yourself struggle a bit. See what comes up: maybe nothing, maybe something. Have another taste, and repeat the process until you feel that you can hold the memory of the taste in your mind, until you can almost taste the whipped cream in your mouth. Try this exercise with different foods to cultivate your taste memory.

Extreme Snacking

habit change   Snacks are fundamentally frivolous and, therefore, don't have to be taken seriously. Use snacking as a form of gustatory extreme sports. When choosing a snack, look for something new to try. So, instead of guiding your snack choices by cost and value, take some chances. There are many foods in this world. Let snacking be a discovery, an adventure, a journey into a land of exotic and unfamiliar tastes! Take your mouth (and your mind, for that matter) to some place it hasn't been before. Visit your local health-food grocery, specialty store, or any ethnic grocery store to look for unique snack foods. If craving a salty snack, for starters, try wasabi-coated green peas; steamed, ready-to-eat edamame soybean pods; vegetarian sushi; roasted nori seaweed. For an adventurous dessert, dare to try chocolate-covered insects (such as water beetles or crickets). Or simply explore such cultural dessert classics as chocolate, strawberry, or almond pocky sticks from Asia or baklava from Greece or the Middle East. To wash down all of this excitement, try a unique and culture-specific beverage, such as, say, a kombucha drink from Asia or kvas from Russia.

Water Study: A Sensory-Linguistic Exercise

 We know the taste of water, but can we describe it? Try, and find yourself at a loss for words. How can such a universally familiar taste be so elusive? One possible explanation is that water doesn't have a chemical taste, just a physical mouth-feel, such as temperature (cold or hot) and the gliding smoothness with which it caresses the mouth. If water tastes salty or sweet, it's salt or sugar that we are tasting, not water. Somehow, when it comes down to water, the word "tasteless" is a compliment, whereas with anything else, it's a criticism. Try three types of bottled water. Which water tastes best? Which water flows best? Which flow is tastiest? What does tastelessness taste like?

The Color of Sweet

 Do you have a favorite sweetener? How did you choose it? Was the basis for your choice cost, family tradition, a rumor about possible health effects, or was it the color of the package? Explore your favorite color of sweet. Our contenders are three artificial sweeteners: Equal in the blue corner, Sweet'N Low in the pink corner, and Splenda in the yellow corner. We'll also use a nonartificial contender, stevia, in the green corner. You will need four teacups and two packages of each kind of sweetener. Empty one package of each sweetener into the trash, and tape an empty package underneath each teacup. Make four cups of tea and sweeten each cup with a different sweetener (put the Sweet'N Low in the cup with the Sweet'N Low package taped underneath, the Splenda in the Splenda cup, and so on). Now shuffle the cups for a blind test. Let the games begin! Sample the cups of tea and arrange them in your order of preference, with your favorite to the left and least favorite to the right. Sip the top two contenders again to ascertain the champion taste. When certain, set the champion sweetener aside and empty the other three cups, turning them over to see which sweeteners fell by the wayside. Drink to the champion sweetener by savoring the rest of the cup. Now you know your favorite color of sweet.

From Start to Finish and Back

awareness While the term *finish* is often used as a measure of wine, few apply it to food. The finish is both an aftertaste and an *afterfeel* (a residual mouth-feel). Take dark mint chocolate, for example. The subtle bitterness you taste is the aftertaste of the dark chocolate, but the breezy cool-ness you feel is a residual mouth-feel from the mint. The finish reveals subtle characteristics of the flavor and may play a deciding role in whether you come back to a given food or not, since the finish is what you're left with after you finish eating. Study the finish as you eat. Has the food left a sweet, lingering, velvety touch or a bitter footprint of astringent gruffness? Time the finish to see how long foods linger invited or uninvited in the doorway of your mouth. Noticing the finish can slow down your eating. Often, after we swallow the food, we consider ourselves to be finished with the bite. But we're not finished with the bite until we've experienced its finish! You can make the experi-ence of eating last by overeating, or you can prolong the experience of taste by studying its finish. With some foods, the finish is the start of the enjoyment.

The "Mmm" Mantra

awareness &
habit change

"Mmm" is a mantra of gustatory enjoy-ment. The "mmm" is the "om" of mindful eating. "Mmm" is the music of savoring. And, indeed, this sound, like no other, celebrates the awareness of flavor. Some eaters appear to amplify their eating experience by making the "mmm" sound as they slow down to savor a particularly auspicious eating moment. Try saying "mmm" to enhance your eating enjoyment, however banal the foodstuff. You can try saying "mmm" out loud or under your breath, before the first bite or after every bite. The chances are that as you "mmm" (to coin a verb) in expectation of enjoyment, you will find yourself being more mmm-mindful of your eating experience. Don't just eat it—mmm it!

The Case of Mayo

awareness In *Blink: The Power of Thinking Without Thinking*, Malcolm Gladwell (2007) writes about the amazingly complex choices our minds make in the blink of an eye, without any conscious processing. Gladwell speaks of professionals who are able to understand, explain, and consciously replicate these intuitive judgments. One such category of professionals is that of food tasters. Whereas most of us will make an overall judgment of preference, expert food tasters are able to articulate their preferences. Consider the case of mayonnaise. Apparently, it is evaluated on no fewer than six dimensions of appearance (color and color intensity, chroma, shine, lumpiness, and bubbles); on ten dimensions of texture (such as how adhesive or slippery it is, or how firm or dense it feels in the mouth); and on fourteen dimensions of flavor, subgrouped into aromatics (for example, whether the mayonnaise has a predominantly egglike or mustardlike flavor), basic tastes (saltiness, sweetness, and so on), and chemical factors (such as whether it creates burning or astringent or pungent sensations). To complicate matters further, every one of these thirty dimensions of appearance, texture, and flavor is rated on a fifteen-point scale! Gladwell notes that "every product in the supermarket can be analyzed along these lines, and after a taster has worked with these scales for years, they become embedded in the taster's unconscious" (182).

Conduct a study of mayonnaise. Sample and analyze three brands of mayonnaise, using the following simplified rating system. Appearance (color, shine, lumpiness, bubbles). Texture (slippery, firm). Flavor: predominant ingredient (eggs, lemon juice, vinegar); predominant taste (salty, sweet, sour); and chemical (burn, astringent, pungent). Don't bother to rate each and every one of these factors on any kind of scale. The goal is to increase your mindfulness by itemizing the elements of flavor in your mouth. When done, select your favorite brand.

Know Your Food Favorites

awareness — What's your favorite food? What makes it your favorite? If you don't know, learn about your favorite flavor combination. Come up with a list of your favorites. Break the list down into subcategories of flavor. For example, by taste (sweet or savory). Check to see if a certain texture (such as creaminess) emerges as a defining theme. Look for the trends of your enjoyment. Ponder the gustatory formula, the sensory secret behind your favorite flavors. Enough with theory; on to practical matters! Sample the top three of your favorite foods or dishes. Did your taste-memory predictions match the reality of your tongue? Can you now answer the question of what makes your favorite food your favorite food? Some things we just have to know precisely!

Start a Food Blog

awareness &
habit change
Try keeping a food blog. First, decide on the scope of your blog. You could do a breakfast blog about cereal brands. Or a blog about new eateries. Or a blog about your tasting club. You could do a cooking blog in which you celebrate your cooking genius or record your culinary misadventures. You could blog about the best convenience-store delis. Or, better yet, you could blog about food blogs. How might this be useful to you? Well, in order to narrate an encounter with food (or anything else for that matter), you have to be mindful enough to encode the experience in your consciousness in the first place. My suggestion: instead of wasting time logging the mindlessly consumed calories, spend some time blogging about what you ate.

Sampling Mini-Fruits, Teas and Tisanes, and Liquid Breads

awareness

Sampling is a great way to cultivate mindfulness of flavor. Here are three sampling suggestions.

Sampling berries. You can think of berries as berries, or you can think of them as minifruits. Did you know that berries are purposefully bright and visually stimulating to attract animals so as to be eaten and, thus, to have their seeds disseminated? What a marvelously histrionic attention-getting scheme! Assemble a tray of various kinds of berries: blackberries, blueberries, cranberries, currants, strawberries, and raspberries. Take a look. What berry calls out to the animal in you? Sample one berry at a time. Study the flavor. Enjoy your mindfulness.

Sampling teas. There's tea and then there's tisane. True tea is made from steeping the leaves of the plant *Camellia sinensis*. Teas, unless decaffeinated, have caffeine and come in four varieties: black, green, oolong, and white. Tisane is an herbal "tea" made from various leaves, roots, seeds, or flowers of such plants as chamomile, dandelion, chrysanthemum, honeybush, and rooibos. Tisane, unless integrated with tea, is caffeine free. Sample a few teas and herbal teas. Compare and note the colors and the aromas. Enjoy your mindfulness.

Sampling nondairy milks. Whereas berries are foods and teas are beverages, milks are beverage foods. If dairy milk is akin to liquid cheese, then grain-based nondairy milk is akin to nonalcoholic beer in the sense that it is like "liquid bread." While I'm sure you know the taste of dairy milk and even the taste of such nut-based nondairy milk as soy milk, you may not be familiar with the wider variety of grain-based nondairy milks. Try out a few "slices of liquid bread" by drinking a glass of oat milk or rice milk. Enjoy your mindfulness.

An Egg Sample of How to Sample Methods of Food Preparation

awareness

It's said that there is more than one road to Rome. Well, most of us haven't meandered enough through Europe to ascertain the former. We can, however, sample more than one way to prepare an egg. As you probably know, eggs can be hard-boiled, soft-boiled, shirred, coddled, poached, fried, scrambled, Benedicted, bedeviled, and whipped into meringue. What a variety of ways to abuse an egg! Get a dozen eggs and call in sick, and then methodically prepare eggs as many ways as you have the patience for. Take in the splendor of the mess and then sample this incredible, edible variety. Don't overdo it: the idea is to sample, not to cover up the evidence of your egg-ocentricity. Compare the flavors. Enjoy your mindfulness. Clean up the mess, refrigerate and/or share the leftovers. On a smaller scale, you can conduct this kind of comparison at any meal by cooking doubles. If you are cooking potatoes, for example, you could both mash and scallop or boil and roast them. This kind of comparison of tastes, as a form of conscious sensory discrimination, is a call to mindfulness. And paradoxically, thanks to a more mindful approach to flavor, by cooking doubles you might end up eating half the amount.

Sampling the Degree of Difference

awareness The *jnd*, or "just noticeable difference," is a psychophysics term that refers to slight but perceivable differences between similar stimuli. Say you are choosing between two brands of milk. All things being equal (percentage of fat and vitamin fortification), can you tell the difference between them? If you can't, then either there is no difference, or the difference between the brands is below your threshold of perception. If, however, you are able to tell the difference between these two brands of milk, how noticeable is the degree of difference? Is it just noticeable or very noticeable? Gladwell (2007) notes that professional food tasters use the Degree of Difference (DOD) scale to quantify such differences. On this 0 to 10 scale, 10 stands for "very different," and lower scores stand for barely noticeable degrees of difference between products. According to Gladwell, two brands of salt-and-vinegar potato chips, Lay's and Wise, have a DOD of 8.

Compare premium and nonpremium brands of various food categories using the DOD scale. Make sure that you are comparing the same products, and not apples to oranges. Ask yourself, how different in flavor are these brands? If your results reveal DOD scores below, say, 3 (with brands having essentially the same flavor), ask yourself, is this just-noticeable difference worth the premium price? Draw your conclusions.

Social Savoring Instead of Social Eating

awareness & habit change Social eating is often mindless eating, since the discussion over the table usually has nothing to do with the food on the table. Experiment with shifting the paradigm from social eating to social savoring. Pick an eatery with a novel cuisine or, at least, an updated menu, and go there with the sole purpose of savoring your food. Find yourself a gourmand partner in crime, someone who is as interested in food as in eating and agrees with the following conversational moratorium: no shoptalk, no stress talk, just food talk.

Tasting Club

awareness &
habit change Social savoring does not have to only involve eating out. It can also mean eating in—by taking on the form of a tasting party. In her book, *Tasting Club: Gathering Together to Share and Savor Your Favorite Tastes*, Dina Cheney provides a step-by-step guide to organizing a tasting club. Cheney offers a structured protocol for what she refers to as "deep-tasting" with the goal of learning about various foods and cultivating your palate and friendships, with minimal cleanup (Cheney 2006, 8). Such tasting clubs are an excellent forum for experience-focused social savoring and are a much-needed alternative to the food-focused smorgasbord potlucks that often turn into socially sanctioned binges. Identify a group of friends who might be more interested in social savoring than in social overeating. Identify three tasting themes (say, chocolates, cheeses, and buffalo wings). Get Cheney's book to read up on the nuances of the tasting sessions and take turns hosting tasting parties.

Tuning In to the Tuning Out

awareness &
habit change Say it's cold outside and you get your winter coat out of storage. You put it on and feel surprised by the weight of it. But after just a few minutes of wearing it, you stop

noticing the sensation of the pressure on your skin. This is called *habituation*, a situation in which we get used to and stop noticing certain reoccurring sensations. Habituation is also known as *neural adaptation* because it is adaptive to conserve our attention span and not waste it on information that has no survival value. As such, habituation also affects eating. This is particularly the case with foods that we eat all the time: no matter how flavorful and stimulating the food is, our minds eventually stop noticing the flavor. Ironically, the process of habituation takes the fun out of our favorite foods. The way it works is that when we know we like the flavor of a particular food, we understandably try to eat it more often. But the more we eat a particular food, the less we actually notice its flavor. In addition to this long-term effect, habituation affects our mindfulness in the short term. As mindful as first bites may be, with each subsequent bite, we tend to lose interest in what we are eating.

If habituation is a mind thief, then you want to practice catching it red-handed whenever it tries to sneak your attention away from eating. To counter habituation, practice the following. Try a new flavor of yogurt. Note the habituation, that is, how your mind begins to tune out the flavor. Pause and refocus on the food: look at it, smell it, taste it, meditate on the flavor. Get into a habit of noticing habituation. Tune in to the process of tuning out.

Mindfulness of Smell

When it comes to eating, smell is an important sense. Aside from its role in appetite regulation, it more importantly tells us about what is edible and what is not, and thus serves as a survival guide.

Edible or Inedible? A Game for Your Nose

awareness To build appreciation for the survival value of your nose and to increase your mindfulness of smell, play a few rounds of the Edible-Inedible Game for Your Nose with a mindful-eating partner. One player, known as the Nose, closes his or her eyes while the other player presents various substances for the Nose to smell to detect what is edible or not. For extra points, you can attempt to guess the substance in front of your nose. Take turns being the Nose, and keep score, if you wish, to make it a lively experience. The winner eats the edibles, and the loser eats the inedibles—just kidding. The winner shares the loot. Tip: to throw off the Nose, assemble a variety of fruit-scented inedible cosmetics or candles, or consider various flowers and plants with edible fragrances, such as blue heliotrope, which, despite its toxicity, is known for its cherry-pie odor.

Smell as a Trigger

As a trigger for eating, smell acts as a gateway drug in the sense of introducing, molecule by molecule, our nose (and then our mind) to the intoxicating promise of eating. Calling smell a "drug" is no exaggeration. After all, smell is chemistry: when we smell a given food, however far away from it our nose may be, we are, in fact, coming into direct contact with the miniscule amounts of that food's particles that have randomly roamed into our nasal passages. So, if I smell chocolate, it means that while there may be no chocolate in sight, let alone in my mouth, there's already chocolate in my nose and on my mind. And, unless steered by a conscious mind, the mouth will blindly follow the nose to the source of the smell.

Anosmia-Ageusia Connection: A Two-Way Street

Taste is primarily smell since the "senses of taste and smell are yoked together phenomenologically" (Dennett 1992, 46), and the smell of food accounts for the lion's share of a food's overall flavor. With this in mind, it stands to reason that loss of sense of smell (*anosmia*) can lead to loss of taste (*ageusia*), which can, in turn, lead to a loss of appetite. I am sure you've noticed that when your nose is stopped up, everything seems to taste … tasteless.

Apparently, this kind of temporary anosmia can be induced on demand. As an appetite-suppressing solution,

Compellis Pharmaceuticals has proposed a nasal spray containing the drug diltiazem, which inhibits olfaction. The company "envisions dieters adhering to a 'puff yourself before you stuff yourself' regimen," according to an article in the *Boston Globe*. Compellis also has proposed a nose-numbing cream to provide the dieter with a "smear before you schmear" weight-management strategy (Krasner 2006, D1). While in some individuals, anosmia leads to weight loss, in other cases, individuals who have an olfactory dysfunction gain weight, as they try to compensate for the anosmia-related loss of taste by eating more (Crawford and Sounder 1995; Duffy, Backstrand, and Ferris 1995).

Anosmia on Demand

awareness — Explore the interplay between smell and appetite by simulating anosmia. You can turn off your sense of smell by pinching your nose with your fingers. Compare how the overall experience of different foods changes with your sense of smell turned off. Try this out with foods or beverages that have traditionally been associated with strong aromas. For example, try having a cup of coffee with your smell turned off. You might also use a preventive nose blockade to cut down on grazing if someone's cooking in the house. If you discover that turning off your nose downregulates your eating to a meaningful degree, you could try throwing off your nose by applying a bit of Vicks VapoRub to the tip of your nose to block food smells. While Vicks VapoRub is a widely used over-the-counter preparation, I do, however, encourage you to clear this experiment with your physician.

Mindfulness of the Movements of Eating

Eating is a complex motor behavior that consists of the coordination of arms, hands, neck, and mouth. The kinesthetic awareness of eating involves monitoring your eating posture, your eating movements, the use of utensils, and the specific kinesthetic signature of the given foodstuff. Becoming more aware of the movements of eating can help you learn to slow down and be more mindful of the eating experience.

Eating Posture

Some eat sitting at the dining table, some eat on their recliners, and some eat on the floor. Some eat standing at a bus stop, some at the kitchen countertop while reading through the classifieds. Some eat lying down with a book. Explore posture for opportunities for mindfulness.

Eating While Sitting on the Floor

awareness & habit change If you are used to eating at the table, try eating while sitting on the floor in a half-lotus, cross-legged position or on your knees with your posterior resting on your heels. You might want to place a tablecloth on the floor. Put on casual clothes that you don't mind staining since eating on the floor might present a bit of a challenge for your hand-to-mouth coordination. Note how this change in posture changes your eating movements. Are you noticing the stretch of your back as you lean forward to pick up or put down a plate? Are you suddenly more cautious as you carry a spoonful of soup to your mouth? Are you less willing to stick around and eat for pleasure because of the increasing discomfort in your knee joints? What about your willingness to get up to get something extra from the kitchen? If eating on the floor helps you feel more mindful, pilot it as a habit for a few weeks. Try this out with the meal that you tend to typically overdo.

Eating While Standing

awareness & habit change Eating while standing is another way to increase the mindfulness of your eating movements. Eating while standing is likely to challenge your sense of balance and, thus, wake up your mind. Sitting down and making ourselves comfortable is a cue for rest and is often an invitation to eat. Eating while standing will help you appreciate the distinction between your need for rest (to sit down, to take a load off) and your need for nutrition, and the ridiculousness of combining these two rather unrelated needs. You might also want to track how the amount of what you eat can be a function of whether you are sitting or standing. Ponder this relationship between your standing and eating stamina. You are likely to discover that when you eat sitting down at a table, you are more likely to try to prolong the pleasure of eating, and to overeat as a result, than when you eat while standing. It's no coincidence that we speak of how much we can eat in one sitting. Oversitting at a dinner table may contribute to overeating, and understanding this may help curb overeating. If you decide to pilot this exercise as a habit, you could choose to stand while snacking or, alternatively, during the meals that you've previously associated with overeating. There's a chance that you will feel satisfied on less food.

La-Z-Boy or O-Bese-Boy?

awareness

Contrast eating while sitting in an upright position (at the dining table or on a couch) with eating while sitting back in a recliner. Ponder how the angle between your legs and your torso contributes to your ability to notice the onset of fullness.

Eating in Bed

Is there anything more annoying in this world than having to get up from the bed to refill your bowl of chocolate chips and nuts when you are all tucked in with a nice book in your hands? I don't think so. But, seriously, do you eat in bed? Do you sleep in a mess of cookie crumbs? Have you taken the breakfast-in-bed idea a bit too far? If so, study your eating-in-bed routine. Do you sit up or lie down? What side do you have your food on, left or right? Or do you keep it on your chest, moving it up and aside when you need to see the bottom of the page? Does eating in bed help you stop shuttling back and forth to the fridge? Or do you still keep popping back up to reload every so many pages? If eating in bed tends to lead to overeating, try, at least for a week, to do your eating at the table.

Eating Movements

Eating movements are probably some of the best-practiced motor behaviors that we have in our repertoire. After all, we've been practicing them since birth. Eating involves perfectly choreographed hand-to-mouth coordination of multiple muscle groups working in flawless unison. In fact, eating movements are so basic that we do them without thinking. To become more conscious of how you eat, try the following exercises.

Shadow Eating

awareness

Like shadowboxing, shadow eating is movement without an opponent: going through the motions of eating without the actual food. Imagine a bowl of soup. Shadow-eat it in real time. Sit down at a table, pick up the imaginary spoon, dip it in the imaginary soup, and carry it to your mouth. Shadow-eat the whole bowl. Note the uncertainty of your movements, the thoughts about whether you are doing it right. Note the tendency to skip the steps of eating or to do them out of sequence. Are you unsure about what to do with your hands between the bites? Isn't it amazing that without the sensory feedback of the actual food and tableware, our minds find it challenging to replicate a series of motions that they have previously performed so mindlessly? Try this with different kinds of food: shadow-eat a hot dog, a bag of potato chips, and a plate of spaghetti.

Eating with Wrist Weights

awareness Whereas shadow eating wakes you up by eliminating the sensory feedback, this exercise will awaken you by distorting the sensory feedback. Put on wrist weights and try eating a few meals with them on. Note a newfound appreciation for the previously ignored precision of your eating movements. Note the difference in your level of mindfulness. Try this out with different weights. Tip: wear casual clothes.

Eating with Your Nondominant Hand

awareness Same idea, different method: try eating with your nondominant hand. Since eating manners vary, and I don't know yours (that is, which hand you hold the knife with and so on), do this: switch everything around from the way that you eat now. Also try to eat with your nondominant hand, while, at the same time, disorienting your dominant hand with a wrist weight. Note the confusion of the mind and an increase in your level of mindfulness.

The Hypnosis of Utensils

Utensils are part of the hypnotic ritual of eating. They cue our hands (and minds) to a certain complex of motor behaviors. As such, a utensil is an ignition key to the mindlessness of eating.

Utensil U-Turn

awareness To this day, some cultures employ their hands instead of utensils for eating. Whatever your opinion of eating with your hands may be, try to do it. Eat a dish—say, rice—with your hands. Get extra napkins. If eating in company, consider having a central bowl for an additional degree of intimacy. Note the new choices you have to make: should you pinch clusters of rice with your fingers and carry it over to your mouth a pinch at a time, or should you use one of your hands as a makeshift bowl, feeding yourself from it with the other hand? Appreciate this new interface of touch between your body and the food, as the skin of your fingers suddenly becomes a new source of information about the heat and texture of the food. Now, if you eat with your hands to begin with, I invite you to a similar utensil U-turn. Experiment with using utensils.

Edible Utensils

awareness & habit change Improvise edible utensils. Use a firm cabbage leaf as a spoon, a sharpened carrot stick as a makeshift skewer, a slice of bread to sponge up your soup, a pair of celery sticks as edible chopsticks. Note the increase in mindfulness as you manipulate food with your improvised edible utensils as well as the joy and satisfaction you receive from field-testing your creativity. Ask yourself, "What healthy food could I use to fashion an edible utensil?" In addition to increasing your mindfulness of the process of eating and sneaking in a few extra servings of vegetables and grains into your meals, you'll have no forks, knives, or spoons to clean up afterward. You'll have eaten them.

Straw Sip vs. Free Sip

awareness & habit change When you drink a milk shake or a smoothie, do you usually sip through a straw or with your lips? Contrast and compare straw sips with free sips (lip sips) the next time you have a liquid food, such as a smoothie or a shake. Divide the glass in half (pour into two separate glasses), and then consume one half through a straw and the other half without a straw. Note the difference in the time it takes to finish each serving. Does it take longer for you to sip through the straw, or do you, on the contrary, suck in the contents faster when using the straw? Does the direct contact of lips with the cold liquid of the smoothie slow you down or do you, on the contrary, tend to chug the stuff down when free sipping? Does using the straw lead to any change of taste as the liquid is being pumped right into the back of the mouth? Does this different delivery to your tongue affect the taste? Do you tend to pace yourself and savor more when drinking through a straw? I am making no particular predictions on this point: examine which kind of sipping leverages the most mindfulness for you. Once you have established the sipping modality that allows you to be most mindful of the flavor, use this knowledge to inform your sipping habits.

Nonutilitarian Utensils

awareness

Utensils provide utility. To refocus on eating, take the utility out of your utensils. As an awareness-building exercise, experiment with unfamiliar utensils. For example, if you are not familiar with the use of chopsticks, try chopsticks. If you generally eat with chopsticks, switch to using a fork. If you are equally adept at using chopsticks and forks, get a set of chopsticks that are unusual in size for you (maybe junior chopsticks or giant chopsticks) to wake up your mind by throwing it off its mindless balance. You could also replace your fork or chopsticks with corncob skewers. Similarly, throw your mind a curveball by increasing the curvature of your spoon: switch to a ladle. Or you could use some of the historical progenitors of modern utensils: arrowheads as knives, seashells and horns as spoons, or tweezers to simulate the old-style two-tine forks (just make sure you sterilize them first).

Kinesthetic Signature

Each food has its own kinesthetic signature, or profile of eating movements. Eating a strawberry is different from eating a steak, that is, if you're mindful.

A User's Guide to Eating Popcorn

awareness

Write a step-by-step guide for eating popcorn. Pop some corn and document your experience. Be precise: skip nothing and specify everything. Make recommendations on how many popcorn clusters to clasp with your fingers to fit the serving into the average-sized mouth without dropping any of the pieces; advise on how to deal with the unpopped kernels. Next, have a friend eat a bag of popcorn per your instructions. Have a laugh. Try this out with different foods. Why? Taking time to narrate an eating experience allows you to become aware of the subtle behavioral eating sequences that have previously slipped your mind.

The Perfect Move: Eating Optimization Exercise

awareness Each food has its own kinesthetic profile, so how can we optimize it? Take spaghetti, for example. You can swirl it around on a fork or cut it up with a knife or lift it up as is and let your tongue pick up the hanging strands. What's the best move? Analyze the kinesthetic signature involved in eating a particular foodstuff, and then try to improve the process by finding an alternative way of eating it. What criterion should you use for deciding that optimization has been achieved? That'll depend on the food. If it's spaghetti, you can judge the move by how often a blob of spaghetti falls back onto the plate so the sauce stains your shirt. If you're spreading cream cheese on a cracker, you can tell by whether the cracker breaks from too much pressure applied to its surface. Granted, this is an exercise for eating geeks. But let's not forget that a defining characteristic of geekiness is presence of mind, albeit in matters of seeming irrelevance.

Becoming Mindful of the Meal Script

Eating as an activity, both at the level of a meal and the level of a bite, is acted out mindlessly in accordance with an over-rehearsed script with the often unhappy ending of overeating. I invite you to examine this conceptual plot and to begin rewriting it.

Rewriting the Script at a Bite Level

At the level of a bite, eating may involve the following seven steps. Once you've decided to eat and what to eat, you next make (1) a decision about what specific part of the dish to eat first. This typically happens without much consciousness. Next is (2) the act of physically manipulating the morsel of food (with or without the utensils). In the case of finger food, you'd go from step (1) to step (3), which is the act of placing the food in your mouth. This may or may not be followed by (4) the act of conscious tasting and savoring of the food. Following and/or in parallel with tasting, you'd proceed to (5) chew the food (which may or may not be conscious). After the chewing, you'd (6) swallow the food, and maybe (7) pause (with or without putting the utensils and/or food down) before the next bite. As you see, each bite is a complex series of steps on a behavioral autopilot that, on the one hand, automates the process of eating and, on the other hand, begets the mindlessness of eating.

It is true that to break down each bite into separate steps is a bit pedantic. But how are we to breathe awareness into a meal without becoming aware of a single bite? Deborah Kesten (1997), in her book *Feeding the Body, Nourishing the Soul*, describes the Buddhist practice of mindful eating: "To experience a meal with a mindful awareness, consider organizing a meal around phases," and "consider that eating is action and sensation" (98–9). With this advice in mind, to rewrite the bite script, to include yourself as a conscious protagonist in this play of life, practice infusing mindfulness into these otherwise mindlessly interlocked seven steps of taking a bite. And you can accomplish this with nothing more than—eating. Kesten advises: "From the start to finish of your meal, your intention is to link the moments together into a continuous stream of sensory awareness" (99).

Just One Bite of Just Eating

habit change You've heard this before: when you eat, just eat. To just eat, and not let your mind wander, is a lot. But why should you just eat and not read a newspaper or watch TV? After all, it's just eating. But it's not just eating! Mindful eating is a commitment to being present; it's eating in real time. As such, mindful eating teaches about the essence of time: time isn't measured in minutes; time is moments, moments of awareness. When unattended, these fleeting moments of our lives are lost from conscious experience, never to be recovered.

Form a habit of starting your meal with just one bite of just eating. Mentally count from one to seven as you hand-hold your consciousness, from deciding to take a bite to identifying what to bite to physically manipulating the food to bringing it to your mouth to taking the steps of tasting and chewing to swallowing, and finally, to pausing. Pause to appreciate this moment of eating as a noteworthy moment of being alive.

Rewriting the Script at a Meal Level

At the level of a meal, most eating episodes are staged to follow the three-act structure of prelude (an appetizer in the way of a soup, a salad, or some finger food), the main act (a main course), and the climax (a dessert). But these acts aren't really acts unless they are mindfully enacted. An act, after all, involves an actor. An act without an actor is a reaction. Add a dollop of mindfulness to your meal to help you change the course of your eating.

Dessert First

awareness What would change about the overall experience of the meal if you had dessert first? Would you then skip the appetizer and not rush through the main course just to get to the dessert, and eat less as a result? Paraphrasing Pink Floyd, why should we, after all, have to eat meat before we can have any pudding? Try eating dessert first a few times to see what, if any, effect this kind of resequencing might have on the state of your mind and body.

Matching Tableware with Food

awareness Consider matching your tableware to the specific dishes you are planning to eat. This might strike you as a bit strange, but strangeness is a precursor to mindfulness. Strange things disrupt the pattern of mindlessness; they awaken our awareness by compelling our attention. Say you were to serve sushi in a kind of tableware you'd find in a sushi bar. The chances are you would, at least initially, attend to the aesthetics of the dish and, thus, also be more likely to attend to the food itself. Aside from trying to re-create the cultural ambience of the dish with culture-specific tableware, you could also think of tableware as a way to complement the appearance of the food. With this approach, you would be testing an artistic hypothesis and, therefore, remain more present during the meal. The bottom line is this: if you spend a moment deciding what plate will look good with the food, you will increase the chance that you will actually look at the food to see if the food does, indeed, look good with the plate you chose. And looking at the food is the beginning of paying attention to the process of eating it.

Becoming Mindful of the Meal Setting

Where we eat and how much we pay for food are just as related to the overall experience of eating as food itself is. Good food in a bad place and bad food in a good place are two very different scenarios. Candlelight and soft music don't make bad wine good, but they do make it better. Eating a sandwich while you are stuck in traffic will help you kill time. Eating the same sandwich after a vigorous mountain hike at a scenic overlook could be a peak experience. The context of the meal determines its experience. Cultivate mindfulness of the settings in which you eat in order to identify the settings that will help you cultivate mindfulness of eating.

Your Favorite Place to Eat

awareness What is your favorite place to eat? List all the types of places and settings where you eat: home (dining room, bedroom, kitchen, laundry room, basement), at work (at the desk, in the cafeteria, at the conference table during meetings), at the in-laws', at a friend's, in bars and restaurants, outdoors (in the park, on the deck, at a drive-in), in various forms of transit (in the car, on the plane, on the train, on the subway, on boats and cruise ships), at buffets, in stores (convenience stores, coffee shops, tea rooms, or when partaking of the free samples at Costco), and so on. Select your all-time favorite place to eat. Go there, eat something, and ponder what you appreciate so much about this particular place and its effect on you. How does this place influence your eating? Does it help you be more mindful as you eat, or does it put your mind to sleep?

Your Favorite Place to Overeat

awareness If you wanted to overeat, where would you want to do it? Do you have a favorite place to overeat? What is it? Your house? Which room? A restaurant, a buffet? A friend's kitchen? Which friend? Your car? What is it about this place that gives you the sanction to ignore all of your good intentions? What makes this place feel so safe? Is it other people overeating around you? Does it give you a sense of invisibility or anonymity? What is the permissive magic of this place? Or is it just a place of habit, a place where you've developed a tendency to overeat? If not sure, go there, eat something, and try to unravel the mystery.

Your Most Mindful Place to Eat

habit change What's your most mindful place to eat? I don't mean a place where you eat well because you feel self-conscious. I mean a place where you're spontaneously conscious enough

119

to eat well and with mindfulness. Do you have such a place? If so, go there to ponder why your meals there come with a side order of mindfulness. While there, meditate on how to turn your favorite place to overeat into your most mindful place to eat. Who knows, maybe they could be one and the same?

Alfresco vs. "Aldesko"

habit change For some people, by choice or circumstance, work is life, office is home, and the desk is the dining table. For others, for whom work is just work, and office isn't home, the desk is still oftentimes the dining table. Whatever you do for a living, chances are that work has become a setting in which you eat. What effect does this have on your eating habits? Have you been eating way too many pizzas and doughnuts? Do you get so caught up in shoptalk that you forget to enjoy the sandwich you brought for lunch? Do you fake healthy eating habits to avoid judgment by your colleagues? If you can, experiment with making a shift from eating "aldesko" to eating alfresco. Compare two workweeks. During the first one, go out to eat during your lunch hour. During the second, stay in.

Now, when I say "go out," I don't mean leaving one building just to enter another. I mean outdoors. Assuming it's not the dead of winter, go on a reconnaissance mission to find your own alfresco eating spots. Come up with a mental map of such spots that are within walking distance of your workplace. Look for nature spots (park benches and picnic tables). Look for spots of interest (promenades or neighborhood basketball courts where, assuming public access, you could watch a pickup game). Also look for a place to hang out. Maybe it's the local courthouse steps you could sit on while you eat, or maybe it's an archway to hide in if it's raining while you snack. Maybe it's a parking deck where, with a sandwich in hand, you can get a bigger picture of the city around you or, perhaps, a glimpse of the sky. Once you come up with this map of alfresco opportunities, go out for lunch for an entire week. Then, the following week, stay in; eat at your desk. Contrast and compare. Make habit-forming decisions.

Eat as If Everybody Were Watching

awareness

Eating is often a public experience, whereas overeating is often done in private. For some, the degree of the public exposure of a meal is an important setting factor and is directly proportional to the degree of mindfulness that accompanies the eating behavior. You've heard the self-affirming advice to "dance like no one's watching." Whereas dancing in private is a harmless undertaking, eating in private, like no one's watching, can lead to overeating. Try eating as if everyone were watching

121

you eat. By eating as if you were in public, your eating will be likely more graceful, and graceful movements require presence of mind. There are several degrees of public exposure you could try. For starters, set up a mirror and watch yourself eat. Or film your eating and review it later with or without company. Finally, you could set up a Webcam and broadcast your eating episodes live. Sounds a bit radical? Well, consider this: self-consciousness is a precursor to self-awareness, and self-awareness is mindfulness.

Car Eating

awareness   Cars are another common setting for our meals. The impact can be quite deadly, from daily laps through nutritionally hazardous drive-throughs to hands-free driving while eating. While a car can be a major hub of distraction, it can also be a perfect sanctuary for mindfulness, however, if parked. In fact, if you are trying to eat alfresco, you will find your car far more private than a park bench unless you double-park on a main street. Go for a brief drive during your next work lunch to find a quiet, scenic spot to park. If the weather is good, lower the windows to get some air moving. Pull the seat back for extra legroom, and mindfully, without rushing, have your lunch. To make your eating experience more serene, and to simulate an even closer approximation of eating alfresco, look for a soundtrack with nature sounds (waves rolling in and out, distant thunderstorms). Or record your own mindful-eating script and play it back while you eat in the oasis of your car.

Caviar in the Backseat

awareness

There is an intriguing interplay between the setting of a meal and our willingness to enjoy it. A dish served in an upscale restaurant will command far more attention than the same dish eaten as a leftover for lunch the following day. A banal slice of baguette dipped into olive oil will evoke more enthusiasm at a restaurant table than it will at the kitchen countertop. Should high-dollar caviar be served in the backseat of a car? "Heavens, no," you may exclaim at the notion of wasting a delicacy on such a prosaic setting. But do we really need the heavily starched linen cloth and the waiter with the endearing foreign accent? Why should the physical coordinates of our eating be such a large factor in our eating experience? Why should we knowingly allow our unconscious to be charmed by the smoke and mirrors of interior-design sophistication when it has nothing to do with the interior of our mouths?

I concede that the setting of a meal can be an ingredient of an eating experience. The sophistication of an eating establishment creates an expectation of quality. This expectation heightens awareness. This heightened awareness becomes a platform for mindful eating. And mindful eating is the best chef. But is it not an insult to our mind that for us to enjoy halfway decent food, we have to be primed to expect it to be great? Is this not a measure of our experiential impotence that we have to rely on presentation to attend to what is already present?

In this exercise, we rebel against the setup of the setting, against the setting up of expectations. We rebel against the elegance and eloquence of these Pavlovian bells and whistles that have conditioned us to expect more out of less. If you can't enjoy caviar or some other exquisite gourmet item in the backseat of your car, throw it away, because you can't enjoy it anywhere. If the backseat of your Ford Taurus is good enough to make love, why is it not good enough to make love to a $250 Fritz Knipschildt dark chocolate truffle? So, what am I proposing here? If you are going to eat well-heeled food, try eating it in the comfort of your flip-flops. Why? To minimize the distraction of the setting and to allow yourself maximum mindfulness to appreciate the exotic taste.

Table Feng Shui: Creating an Eating Place

awareness & habit change Feng shui is the art of creating an optimal living space that is in harmony with its natural setting. In this exercise, create an optimal eating space that is uncluttered enough to accommodate your eating mind. If you have an extra room, try the austerity of an empty room. Let it be your eating room. Let there be only a table and one chair. Avoid doing anything in that room other than eating. If you are confined to the dining table, clean it off before you sit down to eat. Remove any reading matter. The less there is on the table not directly related to your eating, the more room there is for your mind to focus on the food. If the strategy of distraction-proofing isn't to your liking, create an eating space by selecting objects that would cue you to eat mindfully. One way to approach this is by selecting mindfulness-inspiring tableware. The idea of mindfulness as a meditative technology comes from the East. Therefore, you could try using Asian or Asian-inspired tableware as a cue to get into a contemplative state of mind.

Mindful-Eating Placemat: Your Portable Mindful-Eating Space

awareness & habit change Create a mindful-eating placemat. Sketch out a placemat that includes a visual diagram of mindful eating. Draw a picture of the eyes to denote mindfulness of the appearance of the food, with an arrow pointing to a picture of the nose for mindfulness of the smell, with an arrow pointing to a picture of the tongue for mindfulness of the taste. Include various mindfulness callouts such as "Eating Is Movement, Pause the Flow!" or "Mindful, Not Mouthful." A laminated placemat could have taste-recognition check boxes that you could mark off in real time as you study the flavors of your food. In short, create a mindful-eating placemat that you can carry with you like a yoga mat, from table to table, from setting to setting, whether you are eating in or eating out, as a kind of portable eating-mindfulness space of your own.

Developing a Habit of Paying Attention to the Process of Eating

By not paying attention to the process of eating, you miss out on what is going on (1) in your mouth in terms of flavor, (2) in your stomach in terms of fullness, and (3) in your mind in terms of the experience of eating. You end up with a feeling of loss of control over eating and with overeating. This feeling makes sense. After all, control is based on presence of mind—that is, on mindfulness. If you are eating and watching TV, you are either controlling the fork or the remote control; you are either savoring the taste or surfing the channels. You can be either mindful or mindless, conscious or unconscious, in control or out of control. But you can't be both.

To regain control, you have to become conscious of being out of control. In other words, you have to become mindful of being mindless. And that is akin to spontaneous awakening.

Can you count on the eating zombie to wake itself up on its own? Probably not. Therefore, the challenge is to keep the eating zombie from falling asleep in the first place. And this can be achieved by practicing mindfulness of the process of eating to the point where it becomes a habit that kicks in on its own.

CHAPTER 3

Becoming Mindful

of Fullness

Eating is strange. We eat pork rinds but not orange rinds. When on a diet, we don't eat when we are hungry, and when off the diet, we eat when we're not hungry. The reasons we stop eating are no exception to this eating strangeness. Here are just a few:

You run out of the food you like. So you stop eating. If you had the food you like, you'd eat some more, but, oh well.

You run out of time. Not out of food, not out of appetite, but out of time. Back home after a long day at work, you stand in the kitchen grazing and browsing the mail. Feeling guilty about putting your spouse on hold while you "veg out," you promise that you'll be up in five minutes to say good night. And now that the time is up, you gotta go.

You are bursting at the seams. You wish you could eat some more. After all, the reruns of your favorite show are on and it'd be so nice to watch TV and snack, but you just can't. You're really too full. Oh well, maybe you don't want to watch reruns anyway.

The entertainment comes to an end. The show you've been snacking to has ended. With nothing fun to watch, you stop eating, because just eating is boring.

You are "emotionally" full. Now that your stomach is full, you no longer feel empty inside. The tryptophan has kicked in, and you are yawning. Good night.

Your plate is finally clean. Congratulations. Now that you've cleaned your plate, you can put it in the dishwasher to clean it again.

You are overeating and get busted by your partner. Now that your nutritional crime has been witnessed, you stop, not out of fullness but out of shame. "I've had a long day. Can you just get off my case, please!" you protest, slamming the pantry door.

You got your money's worth. Unsure if you got your money's worth, you make a few more trips to the buffet table, dirty dishes mysteriously whisked away by an unseen and permissive server. Heck, you didn't pay eight dollars for just a side salad! But now that your stomach is finally full with value (at least eleven bucks' worth), it's time to leave a three-dollar tip.

When Should You Stop Eating?

When you should stop eating depends on why you are eating at any given time. You have needs to meet, and eating is one way of meeting those needs. If you're eating as a pastime, then eat until you've had enough fun. If you're eating to cope, then eat until you've had enough relief (see chapter 4). If you're eating to connect socially, then eat until you've had enough company. But if you're eating to satisfy hunger, then eat until you've had enough food, that is, until you are full.

A Continuum of Fullness: Three Stopping Points

Assuming you are hungry in the first place, the following three sensations happen after you begin eating. First, the sensation of hunger goes away. This is a moment of *hunger relief*. This happens almost too fast for you to have time to enjoy your meal. If you stop eating at this point, then you no longer feel the painful emptiness of hunger, but you don't yet feel full. If you keep on eating, you will next experience a moment of *pleasant fullness* as the food distends the lining of your stomach, but not so much as to cause pain. If you keep on eating, you will eventually experience a moment of *unpleasant fullness* as the stomach distends to a painful degree.

Why Did You Just Stop Eating?

awareness

Think of the last meal you had. Why did you stop eating? Got full? Are you sure?

Keep a two-week journal using the following list of reasons for eating cessation after each meal:

Hunger relief: You relieved the sensation of hunger.

Pleasant fullness: You reached a point of pleasant fullness.

Unpleasant fullness: You reached a point of unpleasant fullness.

Ran out of food: You stopped eating because the food ran out.

Emotionally felt better: You stopped eating because you felt better inside.

Binge witnessed/shame: You stopped because someone witnessed a binge; you were shamed.

Diet-violation guilt: You stopped eating over guilt about violating a diet.

Entertainment over: You stopped because you had nothing left to watch, read, and so on.

Company left: You stopped eating because you no longer had companionship for the meal.

Ran out of fun food: You stopped eating because you ran out of snacks or fun foods.

Distracted from eating: You stopped because the phone rang or you were otherwise distracted.

Plate clean: You stopped eating because you cleaned your plate or portion.

Got money's worth: At a $12.99 all-you-can-eat buffet, you didn't stop eating until you felt you got a bargain.

Got sleepy: You stopped because you became drowsy or lethargic.

Time up: You stopped because you ran out of time (for example, lunchtime was over).

Ran out of money: You stopped because you were out of money (no change to buy snacks).

Tally the results. What are the typical reasons you stop eating? What does that mean to you?

Zip It

To become more mindful of fullness, tune in to the gradual distention of your stomach as you fill it up with food. Get a gallon-size Ziploc bag. This transparent plastic bag will represent your stomach and will serve as a visual barometer of what's going on in there. Prepare double portions (one for you and one for the bag). As you eat, place an equal amount of food into the plastic bag in front of you. Say you are eating a serving of pasta. When you've consumed a plateful, dump the same amount of pasta into the bag. Notice the plastic bag bulge and expand; notice your stomach bulge and expand. As you chug down a glass of lemonade, pour a glass of lemonade into the plastic bag. Notice the plastic bag bulge and expand; notice your stomach bulge and expand. Having a slice of carrot cake? Dump a slice of cake into the bag. Notice the plastic bag bulge and expand; notice your stomach bulge and expand. To leverage more mindfulness of the gradual distention of your stomach, feed the plastic bag one bite at a time: one for the mouth, one for the bag. Notice the plastic bag bulge and expand; notice your stomach bulge and expand. When done feeding the bag, see if you can zip it!

Celebrate the Moment of Hunger Relief

awareness Assuming clearance from your medical doctor, allow yourself to get a bit hungry, and then eat something to relieve the hunger. Ponder the meaning of this moment; celebrate its primordial universality. Think of the millions of life-forms on this planet, past and present, for which this moment of hunger relief was the ultimate goal, and the accomplishment of this goal was the ultimate biological success. Think of the legions of humans who have perished from starvation, with the unfulfilled dying wish to no longer feel the torture of unrelieved hunger. Think about how in this day of plenty for so many, you are nearly guaranteed not to die hungry. As morbid as this thought might be, rejoice in the knowledge that whatever you will die from, your last moments will most likely be about something existentially loftier and more meaningful than longing for something to eat.

135

Studying the Moment of Hunger Relief

awareness &
habit change
How much food does it take to relieve hunger? Next time you feel the pangs of hunger, have a glass of water. Chances are that the sensations of hunger will be relieved. Don't just take my word for it; see for yourself how the fire of hunger can be put out by a few sips of water! Alternatively, the next time you feel hungry, eat something in the smallest serving possible. Study whether this minimal intervention relieved your hunger. If not, then establish the smallest amount of food needed to relieve hunger. Also track whether there's a relationship between the intensity of hunger and the amount of food necessary to relieve it. You might be surprised to find that your intensity of hunger isn't necessarily proportional to the amount of food you need to relieve it. Hunger operates more like an alarm system than an indicator of how much to eat (Craighead 2006). Just because you're very hungry doesn't mean that you have to eat a lot. So, next time you feel famished, think twice before you order a large pizza. Perhaps a small one will do just fine.

Shoe-Tying Fullness Test

awareness
Tying your shoelaces is a simple way to tell how full you are after a meal. If you've had only enough food to relieve

hunger, chances are you'll be able to tie your shoe-laces without any discomfort. If, however, you are pleasantly, let alone unpleasantly, full, your ability to operate your body might be compromised. The sensations of distress may range from feeling uncomfortable as you squat down to feeling as if you need to loosen your belt before you squat to feeling the bulge of your stomach press against your knees as you squat to feeling short of breath or panting. In the week to come, try the shoe-tying test to check for fullness after you eat.

Pleasant Fullness Essay

awareness

Eat until you feel a pleasant fullness. Circle the words from the list below to describe how you feel.

contented	fulfilled	pleased	happy
comfortable	at ease	satisfied	disciplined
enjoyable	good	easy	relaxed
laid-back	calm	peaceful	stress free
casual	mellow	smooth	placid
sedate	settled	rewarded	on the ball
aware	alert	sharp	capable
competent	sensible	levelheaded	mindful
conscious	thoughtful	nourished	attractive

optimistic	positive	in control	upbeat
certain	clear	confident	constructive
decisive	poised	balanced	controlled
composed	reasonable	well-adjusted	stable
together	organized	unruffled	proper
purposeful	reflective	social	cheerful
complete	whole	lively	active
full of life	dynamic	vibrant	free
appropriate	up on top of things		

Unpleasant Fullness Essay

awareness For the next two weeks, whenever you overeat to the point of unpleasant fullness, circle the words from the list below that are descriptive of your state.

stuffed	swollen	distended	full
overfed	blown up	ballooned	engorged
bloated	satisfied	sated	satiated
dissatisfied	displeased	unhappy	frustrated
disappointed	awkward	ill at ease	clumsy
graceless	bulky	cumbersome	large
massive	mammoth	enormous	bursting
insatiable	gluttonous	voracious	excessive

fat	overweight	heavy	stout
plump	large	corpulent	chubby
big	obese	portly	pudgy
rotund	fleshy	tubby	round
flabby	soft	sagging	chunky
tired	exhausted	sleepy	drowsy
fatigued	worn out	all in	out of breath
drained	pooped	beat	done in
gasping	winded	panting	indigestion
puffy	heartburn	repulsive	bad
nasty	disgusting	hideous	gross
sick	queasy	nauseous	upset
sickening	irritated	annoyed	inert
sluggish	torpid	passive	slow
lethargic	slothful	apathetic	slow moving
gloomy	glum	depressed	melancholic
pessimistic	sad	fed up	despondent
miserable	impulsive	aching	low spirited
undisciplined	tender	sore	out of control
burning	negative	cynical	irritable
touchy	moody	regretful	uncomfortable
wanting to throw up		difficult to maneuver	

The Closure Complex

awareness &
habit change
Some of us grow up with moralizing parents who instill in us an eating ethic of wasting no food. But there's more to the *clean plate syndrome* than just cultural programming. This syndrome, at least in part, has to do with how our minds work with our reliance on the notion of a *category*. Let me explain: when we want something, we want *it* rather than a certain amount of it. When we want a banana, we want its taste (substance) rather than its size or shape (form). At the same time, it's hard for our minds to envision the banana substance abstracted from its form. So, when the mind wants banana substance, it ends up wanting it in the form of a banana. Thus, the thought "I want banana [substance]" unconsciously morphs into the thought "I want a [one whole] banana." As a result, a desire for a taste, mediated by category-driven perception, predetermines the serving size. We see things in units, and we end up eating them in units, forgetting that these naturally occurring units have nothing to do with our physiological needs.

In sum, the mind perceives and consumes in categories. And since a category is a unitary concept, eating only half a banana leaves us with a sense of being unfinished, with a lack of closure. Therefore, when we clean our plates, we do so unconsciously to prevent a sense of lacking closure. It would be odd to think that you had eaten a banana when you know you only had half of it. A half of a banana isn't a banana, after all. So, our decision to stop eating, instead of relying on fullness, becomes a matter of whether we are done eating a particular category of food.

To help you guide your decision to stop eating by considering substance, not form, experiment with rethinking your portion-size decisions. Instead of thinking to yourself that you want an apple (which means a whole apple, a unit of apple fruit), rephrase your desire in terms of the flavor you want. More specifically, try to say to yourself that what you want is not an apple, per se, but a taste of an apple. This way, when having experienced the taste of the apple, you may feel finished even if you are not finished with the rest of the apple.

Fullness, a Bodily Sensation; Satisfaction, a State of Mind

Fullness (also known as *satiety*) fills the stomach, whereas satisfaction pleases the senses. In the search for quality of life, we often confuse satiety with satisfaction. Often, it's only when we satisfy our sensory appetite that we feel that we've finally had enough. The tradition of a dessert at the end of a meal is a perfect example of how we disregard the fullness of the tummy just to experience something yummy in the mouth.

Redefining the Portion Size from Fullness to Mind-Fullness

habit change Portion control, the good old divide (the portion) and conquer (overeating) approach, is not without merit. But what if you redefine the portion size from how many mouthfuls you can have to how many mindfuls you need to feel full, if you shift your attention from a mouthful to a mindful, from a serving to a savoring? What's a mindful? A *mindful*, to coin a term, is a unit of mental absorption in whatever it is that you are doing. For example, as you look back at a typical day, perhaps most of it was spent in a state of robotic, mindless monotony, with the exception of a couple of moments when you were really present, thoughtful, and mindful of something. Maybe you found yourself scratching your head over some challenging problem. Maybe, at the end of your lunch break, you caught a glimpse of a bird swaying on a tree branch. Maybe, when finally home, sitting in your car in the driveway, you had a sense of perspective. Whatever their content, these moments of being mindful are just that: states of being attuned to the moment, absorbed in the here and now. In application to eating, a mindful is a moment of being conscious of eating. Maybe it will last ten seconds, maybe half a minute. But however long, it is a unit of awareness, a serving of mindfulness.

A *savoring*, to coin another term, is a unit of mindful appreciation, a moment of conscious enjoyment, a highlight. To have a savoring, you first have to have a moment of eating consciousness (a mindful). After all, how can you enjoy a moment if you are not aware of it? So, whereas mouthfuls and servings are the units of fullness, mindfuls and savorings are the units of *mind-fullness*.

To help you shift from fullness to mind-fullness, I suggest that at the end of your meals, you look back at your experience and take stock of how conscious you were of your eating and of the moments of eating you enjoyed. How many mindfuls did you have? Which moments were you actually fully conscious? Were you present when you tasted the food? Were you present when you picked up the fork? Were you present when you had a sip of water? How many savorings did you have? Which specific moments of delight did you register? What did you enjoy? Did you consciously enjoy biting into that apple? Did you consciously enjoy the aroma of the bread? Was your mind full? Set a goal: one mindful per serving, one savoring per meal. Challenge yourself, set a more ambitious goal: one mindful per mouthful, one savoring per serving. Shift from the unpleasant fullness of the body to the pleasant expansion of the mind! Redefine "enough."

Speed of Eating and Fullness: The Waiting-Game Solution

While the disappearance of hunger is almost instantaneous after you start eating, the arrival of pleasant fullness takes some time. The less you eat during the time that it takes your stomach to notify your brain that it is full, the less likely you are to overeat. The solution is obvious: slow down.

Pace-Eating: Half-by-Five and All-by-Ten Schedules

awareness & habit change When we eat, we tend to eat the entire portion. This kind of eating doesn't factor in the delay between our stomach's knowing we are full and our brain's knowing we are full. As a result, we overeat by eating beyond the point of pleasant fullness. The following are two pace-eating schedules based on the idea that the more you eat in the first sitting, the longer you should wait before you eat again. *Half-by-five*: divide the portion in half, eat the first half, and then take a five-minute break. If you're still not pleasantly full, eat the remainder of the food. *All-by-ten*: eat all that's in front of you. Wait ten minutes. If still not pleasantly full, have a second helping. For a habit-modifying effect, apply the pace-eating schedule of your choice to the largest meal of the day.

Rest-Your-Hands Technique

awareness & habit change Resting your hands between bites will help you slow down your pace of eating to give fullness time to emerge. Lay down the utensils and rest your hands on the table for ten to twenty seconds. No need to keep track of time. A simple touchdown of your hands on the tablecloth will do. If you eat alone, or are not afraid of coming across as a bit eccentric, try the following. Get two tiny touch bells and put them on each side of the dish. When you rest your hands, you'll hear a ring tone as your hands touch the bells. What shall you do during the pause? Take a breath and listen to the sound fade. Wait to eat another bite until the sound of the bells has faded into silence.

Inverted Eating Race

awareness When eating with a like-minded mindful-eating partner, try to outdo each other in how slowly you can finish the meal. Fill in the pauses with talk. The loser (the one who finishes first) pays the bill. Before you start, say in unison, "Instead of leaving room for dessert, let's leave some room for conversation!"

The Admittedly Annoying Thorough-Chewing Exercise

awareness One of the commonly overlooked phases of digestion is chewing. Chewing takes time, and time facilitates fullness. Conscious chewing is a good way to slow down eating to give fullness time to emerge. Some writers recommend chewing for a certain number of reps, which feels too much like exercise. I suggest you study chewing. What side of the mouth do you chew on? On average, what's your natural number of chewing motions per bite? What's it like to have food in your mouth and not chew, just letting it sit there for a moment? How do you decide when you have chewed enough and that it's time to swallow? Let's chew on that for a couple of weeks.

Slow-Eating Record

awareness Buy a bag of Hershey's Kisses. Take one out. Dump the rest into the trash. Now that you have only one Hershey's Kiss, make this kiss last. Make love to it the way you would to the lips of a parting partner. Kiss it good-bye. Let your tongue do a slow dance, gradually unlocking the nuances of the flavor. Of course, you can't always freeze-frame in this type of gusto-sensual reverie when you eat. But, at least set the record straight: you can slow down when you choose to.

Counting the Chips

awareness & habit change How long does an average bag of chips last when you are vegging in front of the TV? How long is it before your fingers run into the disappointment of broken-chip fragments at the bottom of the bag? Try something different: count the chips. First look at the bag of chips and predict how many chips there are inside. Then count the chips as you eat them. If you don't finish the bag, jot down the number you ate on the outside and continue counting when you come back to this bag of chips during your next snack attack. Compare the actual results with your prediction. Even if the chips are fewer than anticipated, the experience of counting them will certainly help you slow down and prevent a sense of disappointment. Apply this counting tactic to other finger-food snacks and sweets. For example, guess how many raisins or almonds you'll find in a particular bag of trail mix. Count them up or risk inhaling countless calories without a sense of fulfillment.

Reminiscence Eating

awareness Eating links us to people, places, and things of our pasts and, as such, can be a great way of going down memory lane on a journey of self-remembering. *Reminiscence eating* is an opportunity to turn a simple act of eating into an existentially meaningful experience, with the added advantage of slowing down the process of eating and thus giving fullness time to emerge. Next time you eat, look at the food in front of you and allow yourself to free-associate about the past. What does this dish, this smell, this taste remind you of? Give yourself a taste of the past and turn what could have been mechanical and meaningless into something sentimental and mindful.

A Cooling-Off Period

awareness Think of the times you've burnt your lips on a bowl of soup. Isn't it amazing that we are in such a rush to eat that we are willing to burn ourselves?! Next time you have a bowl of soup in front of you, give it a few moments to cool off. Stir it mindfully, watching the vortex of colors swirl. Gently blow air on it, unlocking the aroma. Look around. Enjoy the wait. Exhale the impatience. Chill.

Preloading on Smells, Liquids, and Umami

Preloading can be viewed as an attempt to manipulate fullness and to prevent overeating. While preloading on liquids may feel like a pointless trade-in of liquid-food calories for solid-food calories, preloading on smells as a means to prevent overeating seems like a win-win proposition. A. R. Hirsch (1998) showed that smelling food before eating facilitates fullness and reduces how much we eat. Hirsch also concluded that the brain correlates the amount of aroma we inhale with the amount of the food we take in. Apparently the more you smell the food, the less of it you'll eat. Sound too good to be true? Put your nose to the test.

Noseful-Not-Mouthful

habit change Active, conscious smelling of food facilitates a faster onset of fullness (Hirsch 1998). Try a noseful-not-mouthful approach to preload on the smell before loading up on the food. A practical tip: in addition to washing your hands before you eat, consider also clearing out your nose. Try increasing the ratio of nosefuls to mouthfuls. Whereas before, you'd smell the food just once at the beginning of a meal, see if you can build up to a one-to-one noseful-to-mouthful ratio, in which you make a point to smell the food before each and every bite. Or, at least, try to take a few mindful nosefuls of the food at the beginning of your meal and in between courses.

Soup-erior Fullness

awareness & habit change

In regard to preloading on liquids, J. Fuhrman (2003) advises against liquid calories without fiber, noting that despite their caloric content, they are unlikely to facilitate fullness. Hirsch (1998) notes that hot meals give off more of an aroma than cold dishes. With these points in mind, a warm, fiber-rich vegetable soup would seem like a perfect way to explore whether preloading holds water or not. Compare two appetizers: soup versus an amount of french fries of approximately the same caloric content. What fills you up more? Experiment with preloading on soups to see if doing so can help you eat less of the main course.

Umami: Taste of Fullness

awareness

According to Marcia Pelchat, a sensory psychologist from Monell Chemical Senses Center in Philadelphia, if you add monosodium glutamate (MSG), yellow coloring, and salt to boiling water, "you can make people think they're eating chicken broth." This is the notoriously elusive *fifth taste* of umami, also described as a taste of fullness with a hearty and meaty mouth-feel. Umami is owed to the cells of the tongue that respond to MSG in protein-heavy foods and is enhanced by aging, fermentation, curing, and ripeness (Fletcher 2000).

Whereas so far I have described fullness as an essentially physical phenomenon resulting from the distention of the stomach, umami offers an intriguing possibility of preloading on chemical fullness. Experiment with manipulating your overall experience of fullness by having a cup of that proverbial chicken soup with a splash of soy sauce to augment the umami taste. In so doing, you will be preloading your fullness on liquid, smell, and on umami. Taste the fullness.

Sensory-Specific Satiety

The tongue is a thrill seeker. As it tires of one taste, it looks for another. This sensation-seeking tendency of the tongue is what accounts for so-called sensory-specific satiety. Recall what happens in a buffet: while you may feel too full to eat another plate of roast beef and mashed potatoes, you wouldn't mind trying something else. Sensory-specific satiety makes evolutionary sense: it assures that our food intake is varied in nutrient content. From a weight-management standpoint, however, this insatiable search for novel gustatory sensations entraps us in the horn of plenty, leading us to overeat to a point of unpleasant fullness. Research shows that increased variety of foods, particularly with high palatability, may contribute to development and maintenance of obesity (Hetherington and Rolls 1996; Raynor and Epstein 2001).

Exploring Sensory-Specific Satiety

awareness &
habit change

Sensory-specific satiety is an overeating liability, but there are ways to manage it. Try to remain conscious of whether you're eating to satisfy your biological hunger or sensory hunger. Ask yourself, "Do I want this food because I am still hungry, or am I just interested in its taste?" If chasing the taste, then just taste; have a mindful bite. You don't have to eat a whole serving just because you are interested in a taste! Also, factor in sensory-specific satiety by cutting back on portion size. Leave room for the curiosity of your tongue. In sum, when faced with a diversity of tastes, choose to taste all you can taste, not necessarily to eat all you can eat! Rethink buffets, potlucks, and other kinds of smorgasbords as gustatory galleries. Peruse, don't abuse.

Being Stuffed Doesn't Have to Mean Weight Gain

Strange as it may sound, having a full, even unpleasantly full, stomach doesn't have to mean weight gain. Foodstuffs differ in their caloric density. Having a stomach full of cheese is different from having it full of spinach. Some nutritional authors free their readers to eat as much as they please as long as what they eat is low in caloric density. J. Fuhrman (2003) challenges us to eat at least two pounds of vegetables a day, four pieces of fruit, a cup of beans, and small amounts of nuts and whole grains. Bottom line is that it's okay to overeat, that is, to eat beyond the sense of pleasant fullness, as long as what you overeat is low in caloric density.

Safe Overeating

awareness & habit change If you are shopping for a hassle-free philosophy of eating, and resent portion control and calorie counting, you can overeat and not bother with being mindful of fullness, as long as you mindfully choose what you mindlessly overeat! Fuhrman, the author of *Eat to Live*, couldn't be any more blunt about this: "Completely rethink what your idea of portion control is; make it huge" (2003, 178). So let's overeat! Put together a huge, preferably organic, salad (go easy on the dressing though), turn on the TV, and "veg out." Don't worry about being mindful of fullness. Let your stomach stop you when you are pleasantly or even unpleasantly full. Sound scary? Take solace in the fact that you've already survived this very fear time and time again in your years of overeating. This time, though, you are practicing safe overeating.

Preventing Hunger by Maintaining Fullness

When you eat and fill up, you begin to feel fuller, less hungry, satiated. This active, in-the-moment fullness can be recognized through the pleasant or not-so-pleasant distention of your stomach. You are not just not hungry; you are full. Okay, say it's now been a couple of hours since you ate. Your stomach is no longer distended and you no longer feel actively full, but you also are not necessarily hungry. You are content, neither hungry nor full. This state can be thought of as *fullness*, *satiety*, or, less scientifically, *staying power*. Different foods have different fullness/satiety values. Some foods tide us over for longer periods than others. S. H. Holt has introduced the so-called Satiety Index, which is a rank-ordering of foodstuffs by their ability to keep us from feeling hungry (Holt et al. 1995). Foods high in fat, such as chocolate, have a relatively short-term satiety, whereas foods that are high in fiber, such as beans, have long-term satiety. Both a mindful eater and a mindless eater, when hungry, are driven by a goal of attaining fullness, that is, relieving hunger. A satiety-savvy eater, however, may be driven as well by a desire to prevent future hunger by maintaining a state of fullness through a selection of foods with a high Satiety Index value. Therefore, a satiety-savvy mindful eater approaches a given meal not only from the position of meeting the immediate, tactical needs of satiety but with a strategic long-term view of the progression of satiety over time and how it fits in with a daily agenda and energy demands.

Making Fullness Last

awareness & *habit change* It's a weekday morning and you are wondering what to have for breakfast. A satiety-savvy eater, aware of the fact that some foods have more staying power than others, might have some shredded wheat and bran cereal for breakfast. A satiety-naïve eater would load up on the traditional breakfast fare in a mistaken assumption that the more calories he or she eats, the longer he or she can maintain a sense of fullness. This is likely to boomerang: the high-calorie, high-fat, low-fiber breakfast may spike blood sugar levels, thus leading to a premature onset of hunger. Experiment with making the fullness last. Read up on the Satiety Index and compose breakfast menus with marathon staying power that can help you last through lunch without experiencing intense hunger. Are you, as a result, less prone to snack in the midmorning? Are you less starved at lunchtime? Consider when else during the day you might benefit from such a meal. Perhaps a bedtime snack to keep you from a midnight trip to the fridge? In sum, consider your energy needs and plan your fullness strategically.

Committing to a Definition of Fullness

So, how should you define fullness from this point on? As hunger relief or pleasant fullness? Here's a position of balance: use different definitions for different meals. For example, stop eating breakfast and lunch at the point of hunger relief, and stop eating dinner at the point of pleasant fullness. Workday breakfast and lunch are instrumental in nature. Thus, shift the focus from enjoyment to your energy needs. At dinner, however, make room in your stomach for a bit of pleasure; eat until pleasantly full. Or decide to never eat past pleasant fullness except for on special occasions—holidays, parties, family reunions, or whatever that might be for you. Commit to a definition of fullness that both prevents overeating and preserves the quality of your life.

CHAPTER 4

Mindful Emotional Eating

Here's a taboo thought: eating to relieve stress works! If the strategy of eating to cope didn't work, we wouldn't have a problem with abusing it. What doesn't work, however, is overeating when stressed. Sure, it'd be optimal to never have to use food to cope. But in the meantime, as you work on this long-term goal of food-free coping, approach your habit of emotional eating with compassion. Before you try to give up emotional eating altogether, learn to make better use of this coping strategy by becoming a more mindful emotional eater. Emotional eating isn't a problem: mindless emotional eating is!

How Did Chicken Soup Become the Remedy for the Soul?

How have we come to link foods with moods? Why does eating when stressed seem so intuitive? In fact, eating (not overeating) as a coping response to stress makes good behavioral and physiological sense.

Eating as a Learned Form of Coping with Stress

Here's some irony for you: while we've been socialized to cope with stress by eating, reactive eating enjoys no social sanction. From day one, feeding has been a default parenting intervention, and the pacifier (in all its oral symbolism) has been our first coping tool. To confuse matters further, many cultures explicitly equate feeding with caring. So why is it okay to show your care for others by feeding them but not okay to show your care for yourself by self-feeding? Finally, we keep downloading psychological software of dinnertime as family time, conditioning ourselves from one generation to the next to see eating as a family ritual, as a time of togetherness, as an opportunity for social relating and belonging, as a means to emotional well-being. Give yourself permission to eat to cope! Don't worry; it's the lack of permission that turns emotional eating into emotional overeating.

Eating as a Grounding Ritual

Eating is a ritual, and as such, it is comforting in its predictability. Also, eating is a sensation-rich, unambiguously physical activity. Eating is thus an effective reality check at a time of uncertainty or confusion, a behavior that grounds and centers a suffering mind. Therefore, to maximize the coping usefulness of emotional eating, we have to make emotional eating more ritualized, more systematic, with clear start and end points.

Eating as a Parasympathetic Activity

From the physiological perspective, a choice to eat can be seen as an attempt to directly manipulate the nervous system, by switching on the part of our wiring that is associated with relaxation and rest. You see, the autonomic nervous system (ANS) of your body consists of the *sympathetic nervous system* (SNS), which is activated during stress and prepares the body for fight or flight, and the *parasympathetic nervous system* (PNS), which is responsible for conservation of energy and rest. A choice to eat can be seen as an attempt to turn on the PNS. While eating has been associated with increases in PNS activity (Uijtdehaage, Stern, and Koch 1992), the mere act of mindless eating in and of itself is unlikely to turn on the PNS when you are stressed. But mindful, conscious eating might. So as you eat to cope, smell and taste your food to assure maximally prompt activation of the parasympathetic relaxation response.

Five Principles of Mindful Emotional Eating

To summarize, you have two options in regard to emotional eating: you can try to eliminate it altogether, or you can try to make better use of it by making emotional eating more conscious. The latter would be consistent with the goals of *harm reduction*, a humanistic form of psychotherapy that offers a pragmatic risk-reduction approach to managing problematic behaviors (Marlatt 2002b). The following five principles will help you move from mindlessly reactive emotional eating to mindfully conscious emotional eating in moderation:

1. When eating to cope with emotions, accept emotional eating as a legitimate coping choice, not a coping failure.

2. When eating to cope, first activate the parasympathetic response through relaxation.

3. When eating to cope, whenever possible try to do so in company, not in hiding.

4. When eating to cope with emotions alone, follow a predictable eating ritual, with clear start and end points.

5. When eating to cope with emotions, remember that emotional eating does not have to mean emotional overeating.

Following these guidelines will help you approach emotional eating with a sense of control.

Relaxation as the First Course

habit change The very idea of emotional eating is emotional self-regulation, a return to a baseline of reasonable calmness with the help of eating. To assure maximum emotional gains (rather than weight gains) from emotional eating, use relaxation as a prelude to an emotional eating self-help intervention. I recommend that you begin any of your emotional eating meals with a course of breath-focused relaxation. Doing so will not only allow you to leverage maximum parasympathetic (relaxation) response from your emotional-eating self-help intervention but will also assure optimal digestion of whatever you eat when you eat to cope.

Feeling Verklempt? Talk Amongst Yourselves

habit change Emotional eating doesn't have to be a dirty little secret. When feeling emotionally upset and considering emotional eating as a coping intervention, try to find a supportive companion. Whether in person or by phone, let such a person know of what you are trying to do. Explain that you are upset, that you'd like to talk about it—over food. Show your hand: explain that while you are not exactly hungry, you'd like to supplement comfort food with the comfort of supportive company. If your companion isn't interested in eating with you, that's okay, as long as he or she is willing to just sit with you, without judgment, as you take your time to snack a bit. Explain that you are not necessarily looking for therapy or advice, and you are not looking for someone to solve your problems but just for someone to be with you to process what's going on. Tip: before sitting down with your friend, think about whether or not you want your friend to help you avoid overeating. Clarify to what extent you want him or her to be involved in monitoring your food intake. Thank your friend for being with you.

If you find yourself on the other side of this intervention, in the role of support, do your best to avoid being judgmental of emotional eating. If you feel that the emotional-eating episode is gradually becoming an episode of emotional overeating, remind yourself that you are not responsible for the other's eating behavior. Remember that your presence at the coping table is not a permission to overeat or enabling but a generous offer of support. Tip: before agreeing to be there, ask your friend if he or she wants your help in slowing down and avoiding overeating. Ask, "Hey, I'd love to be there with you as you take care of yourself. Do you want me to encourage you to slow down a bit and remind you not to overdo?" If yes, then do. If no, then just be there for the other person without judgment. This kind of discussion of expectations can help both of you avoid any awkwardness.

State Your Expectation

awareness & habit change When you take a pill for a headache, you have an expectation that it will make your headache go away. It's the same with emotional eating: it's based on your expectation that either the food itself and/or the process of eating will help you feel better emotionally. Try the following the next time you decide to cope by eating: Before you actually eat, write down how you feel and state your expectations of relief. Use the following formula for this exercise: "I am feeling _____ [fill in the blank], and I expect this _____ [describe the given comfort food] and the process of eating it to make me feel _____ [fill in the blank]." Do this for a few weeks. After some time, you might have a collection of statements that look as follows: "I am feeling bored. I expect this bowl of ice cream to entertain me." "I am feeling rejected. I expect this box of crackers to help me feel more okay about myself." "I am feeling really sad, and I expect these egg rolls and cheesecake to help me feel less sad." Take a moment to ponder whether these foods and the process of eating them have, in fact, fulfilled your expectations of relief. If so, great! If not, still great. After all, the more you know about how you are feeling and how you want to feel, the more you know about yourself. And if it takes emotional eating to help you know how you feel and how you want to feel, then, as far as I am concerned, these are calories well spent.

Know Your Comfort Foods

awareness Emotional eating is often haphazard. Do you know your comfort foods? Or do you just rummage around stuffing yourself with foods that don't do anything for you until you find something that actually hits the spot? To help reduce emotional overeating due to random grazing, explore which foods have a sentimental value for you. These "chicken soups" from the past are nutritional placebos that we've come to associate with comfort from the early days of our lives. What are those family feel-good classics that you are still in a habit of serving to yourself when feeling blue? What feelings do these foods evoke in you? Explore your favorite textures. Explore your favorite finger foods. Catalog and understand the comfort foods that work for you. Take the guesswork out of coping.

Normalizing Your Relationship with Comfort Foods

habit change What will you do with all the information about your comfort foods that you gleaned from the previous exercise? Well, now that you know what you crave in times of stress, stock up on it. Not having your comfort foods on hand inadvertently bans them and renders eating them a sin. Alternatively, having easy access to your comfort foods allows you to normalize and legalize your relationship with these foods as coping tools and allows an apple to be an apple rather than a forbidden fruit to binge on. Designate a separate place for these foods. Label it "medicine cabinet" or "toolbox" to remind yourself of these foods' therapeutic and instrumental functions. If you find yourself eating up your comfort foods in the first day or two, consider this the honeymoon phase of your desensitization project and promptly replenish your supplies. Use a craving-control strategy as needed. Finally, dare to coexist with these comfort foods for at least a month.

Sometimes "out of sight, out of mind" works just the other way around: because something is out of sight, you can't get it off your mind. Dare to explore the mechanism of desensitization, which works just the other way around: if in sight all the time, then it's out of mind.

Calibrating the Dosage

habit change If food is medicine, overeating is over-dosing. In the weeks to come, when you feel the need to rely on emotional eating to cope, use these moments as an opportunity to fine-tune the dosage of your comfort foods. Use a stack of yellow sticky notes as your prescription pad. After you have made a conscious choice to cope by eating, write down a prescription for yourself. For example: "Rx.: one serving of ice cream" or "Rx.: ten chocolate-covered almonds." Then, take your emotional pulse: Rate the intensity of your feeling before you treat yourself to your food cure. Then administer the food "medication" and reassess your emotional pulse to see if your expectations of relief were met. Do you still feel bad, or are you better? Do you feel you need another dose? How much do you think will suffice? Are there any side effects? Did you overdo it (did you overeat)? The bottom line is that if you plan to use comfort foods to cope, you have to establish an effective dosing schedule (which is, of course, likely to also vary by food).

Document what works and in what amounts, so you can prevent emotional overeating in the future.

If Food Is Your Therapist, Then Talk to It

awareness & habit change Talking about what bothers you can be cathartic, whether or not you have an audience. Additionally, talking about why you are upset allows you to process the emotional material and crystallize what you need to feel better. Contrary to the title of this exercise, I am not encouraging you to talk to the food, per se, but to talk about how you feel before you engage in emotional eating. Get a handheld recorder and make a point to orally document what's going on for you before you orally cope with it. Once again, do this only if you have first made a conscious decision that you will cope by eating (whether it's because you've tried to cope otherwise and it didn't help or because you just did not feel like coping in any other manner). Start the recording by saying, "I have reviewed my coping options and decided to cope by eating. But before I start coping by eating, here's what's going on for me right now." When you are finished describing what you feel and how you want to feel, administer the food cure. Turn the recorder back on and talk about whether your emotional eating intervention helped or not. Review your recordings for additional insights.

Emotional Eating Koans

awareness A koan is a kind of question used as a training device in the Buddhist tradition, designed to help the student attain a degree of clarity.

Meditate on the following emotional eating koans for additional insights:

Emotional Eating Koan 1: "Who ate my happiness?"

Emotional Eating Koan 2: "When you have a gut feeling, where do you have it?"

Emotional Eating Koan 3: "How many Hershey's Kisses does it take to feel kissed?"

Emotional Eating Koan 4: "What is your mind full of when you feel empty?"

Emotional Eating Koan 5: "Does food have a taste when it is eaten without awareness?"

Ritualizing Emotional Eating

habit change Habits, routines, and rituals offer a soothing, stabilizing sense of predictability and help us feel in control of the moment. Emotional-eating episodes are often haphazard and unstructured. To help you rely less on food and more on the activity of eating during your emotional-eating episode, I encourage you to ritualize and structure your emotional eating protocol. I encourage you to always begin by stating to yourself (out loud or internally) that you are making a conscious choice to cope by eating and that in doing so, you are giving yourself permission not to feel guilty or disgusted with yourself afterward, since emotional eating is, however imperfect, a viable form of self-care. Remind yourself to treat, not judge. After making this statement of intent and giving yourself the permission to cope by eating, identify how you feel and what you are trying to cope with. You might follow this by stating your expectations of how you wish to feel after you eat. Then, consciously consider what you will eat and decide on a "dose." Then, with mindfulness of the process of eating, eat the food. Take your time to savor and appreciate the flavor of the food, as well as the subtle changes in your state of mind and body. Pause to check whether you have attained a desired emotional state; if not, proceed with another serving and check again. When you feel you have attained a desired state (whether you use psychological or somatic/physiological markers for that), allow yourself the realization that you have once again been able to successfully self-soothe with food. Congratulate yourself on another coping success.

Developing a Reminder Mantra for Mindful Emotional Eating

habit change The verb "to treat" can be a useful mnemonic that captures the central point of this chapter and the principles outlined previously. More specifically, this verb offers us a trio of relevant meanings. "To treat" means to care, to heal, to cure, to alleviate, to soothe. "To treat" also means to indulge, to play, to enjoy, to savor. And "to treat," if spelled out as "to tr-eat," turns out to have a built-in "to eat," which is, coincidentally, the point of emotional eating: treating (healing/helping) yourself by eating. With these three therapeutic meanings in mind, I invite you to rethink emotional eating as an opportunity to treat yourself at a time of emotional distress with the help of eating in moderation but without judgment. Or, to put it in a mantra form: "Tr-eat; do not judge!" Use this mantra as is, or spend some time formulating your own mindful emotional eating catchphrase.

Let's Regress

awareness & habit change The comfort of food is not an illusion; it is a psycho-physiological reality. Physiologically, eating is pleasurable: it relieves the pain of hunger and caresses the senses. Psychologically, eating is a time-tested self-therapy that we were taught by our parents and caregivers when they comforted us by providing access to a mother's breast, a bottle, or a pacifier. As such, emotional eating can be viewed as a kind of developmental regression to an arguably unsophisticated level of coping. But we don't have to feel ashamed of that. One aspect of emotional maturity is the ability to self-soothe. And you already know how to do that in a variety of ways, even if one of them is by eating. However, we all function through a range of coping techniques, some days getting by on just the wisdom of self-talk and on other days needing something a bit more heavy duty.

So, instead of fretting about your coping imperfections, go ahead and regress a bit! You will need the following supplies: a set of comfortable pajamas, a blanket, and a good book. With these supplies in stock, the next time you decide to cope by eating, regress: curl up on the couch with a good book and tuck in the blanket. Allow yourself to get cozy and do that forbidden thing that your parents told you never to do (eat and read in bed). Try this recipe for regression, or create and experiment with your own. In short, I invite you to embrace your regressions, not as retreats, not as surrenders but as a rational falling back, a return to the previously dug trenches of simplicity, to recoup before you return to the battlefields of adult life. And by maximizing the regression of the emotional eating factor, you just might minimize the amount of food you need to get the coping value you crave.

Harm-Reduced Hand-to-Mouth Trance

habit change Emotional eating is regressive, no doubt about it. And that's okay: even adults need their pacifiers from time to time. Finger foods (such as chips, popcorn, nuts, candy, crackers) make good pacifiers. Unlike, say, a sandwich, finger foods have the advantage of lasting. It's almost as if by opening a bag of potato chips or a bag of M&M's, we guarantee ourselves the continuity of pleasure. The oblivion with which we plow through boxes of Triscuit crackers or bags of tortilla chips seems to quell our racing minds by putting us in a kind of soothing trance of hand-to-mouth self-feeding.

Appreciating the relaxing value of this self-feeding trance allows us to optimize the cost-to-benefit ratio of emotional eating. All we have to do is to keep the trance while minimizing the caloric intake. How? By substituting unhealthy finger foods with healthier finger foods. Now, let's be realistic: if you are reading this book, a bag of baby carrots will probably not do. But some substitutions can certainly help you reduce the damage of this kind of mindless vegging. If hand-to-mouth emotional eating is a staple of your coping, I encourage you to make a conscious shopping choice to stock up on frozen berries of various sorts, and, when necessary, plow through a bowl of those. This way, you are likely to sow fewer unwanted calories. Let alone, this type of finger food is healthy for you anyway. Also, to give the trance enough time to set in, slow down your eating by taking only one piece of finger food at a time. This way, even if you are feeding yourself an unhealthy, calorie-rich finger food, you can make it last longer and thus prevent emotional overeating. More specifically, retrain yourself to have one chip, candy, nut, or popcorn cluster at a time. Experiment with these modifications to get more trance per calorie from your emotional eating.

Maintaining Mindfulness During an Emotional-Eating Episode

habit change By maintaining mindfulness during an emotional-eating episode, you can prevent it from becoming a runaway train of emotional overeating. Following are a few tips for how to maintain a degree of mindfulness as you cope by eating.

Use your nondominant hand: Eating with your nondominant hand is a more mindful eating experience, since doing so feels awkward and unfamiliar, and therefore requires some supervision from your mind. The more mental supervision you can allocate to eating, the less you will eat.

Use a utensil: The use of utensils requires some degree of psychomotor concentration, which will help you remain more mindful of the overall eating process.

Dress up or stay dressed: Stay dressed if you've come from work, since your clothes (belts, waistlines, buttons) serve to amplify the distention of your stomach and will help you stay alert to the onset of moderate fullness so you can avoid reaching a point of uncomfortable fullness. Alternatively, change into something nice, such as your favorite shirt or blouse, to force yourself to remain mindful enough of your eating to avoid ruining a favorite piece of clothing.

Introduce a random object: Take a grocery bag, put a pair of sneakers inside, and put it on the table. Why? Why not! Sure, a pair of sneakers doesn't belong on the dining-room table. But, you know what? Right now this eating table is not really a table but a coping workstation, and this bag of sneakers just might help you stay awake enough to not gorge on a bag of Snickers bars. As an emotional eater, you already know that emotional eating is not about food anyway!

Reframing the "What-the-Heck"

habit change

One way an otherwise innocuous emotional-eating episode morphs into an emotional-overeating episode is through the miracle of "what-the-heck" rationalization. I am sure you know what I mean: you realize you've eaten more than you would've liked and you think to yourself, "Well, I blew it. What the heck! I might as well keep on eating." Let's face it. "What the heck" and "might as well" functionally mean nothing less than "screw my goals"! Here's what I'd like for you to do: take a sheet of paper and write down the following equation twenty times: "what the heck" = "screw my goals."

Overeating vs. Binge-Eating

Binge-eating is a form of overeating that is typically characterized by eating an objectively large amount of food and by an accompanying feeling of loss of control. While this definition makes theoretical sense, in practice establishing what constitutes an objectively large amount of food, let alone what constitutes a feeling of loss of control, can be quite difficult. It should be noted that binge-eating is emotional eating in the sense that it is an attempt at emotional self-regulation, motivated by a desire to change how you feel. But traditional emotional eating and binge-eating have somewhat different emotional goals. The goal of traditional emotional eating is to return to the emotional baseline, from feeling distressed to feeling normal. The goal of intentional binge-eating is to numb out, to feel nothing.

With this in mind, a mere runaway emotional-eating episode is not actually a binge. It's just a lapse of mindfulness. For an overeating episode to be a true binge, you'd have to more or less knowingly pursue the goal of an altered state of consciousness; you'd have to want to eat yourself into a state of oblivion. Why is this important to understand? Well, the way I see it, mindfulness is fundamentally incompatible with a state of oblivion. In other words, there is no way to infuse a degree of mindfulness into a binge without defeating the purpose of the binge. What this means is that if you want to binge to the point of oblivion, all you can really do to make it more psychologically healthy is to give yourself conscious permission to do so in order to prevent the post-binge regret that might trigger unhealthy compensatory behaviors or another binge. You can also postpone the binge.

Postpone the Binge

habit change

Let's suppose that you've had a truly awful day. You are at your wit's end: you've tried every coping strategy you know and you still feel bad. Or, perhaps you are so fried that you made a decision that you are going to binge—not just eat to cope in moderation but to go all the way—until you feel really stuffed and numb to everything inside and outside of you. What can I say other than that I am sorry that you feel so bad that you need to lose yourself to make it through another day? And there may be more days like this. In addition to giving yourself the conscious permission to go ahead and proceed with the binge (in order to minimize the post-binge regret that might trigger unhealthy compensatory behaviors and/or another binge), you can also try postponing the binge by a few minutes. While you wait, consider if, perhaps, you could be satisfied with an emotional-eating episode instead of a binge. If you decide that an emotional-eating episode will not cut it for you, then proceed with the binge. If, however, you conclude that an emotional-eating episode might actually do it for you, then attempt to have a mindful emotional-eating episode using the damage-control strategies suggested in this chapter. Challenge yourself to eventually extend the delay from, say, five minutes to ten or fifteen minutes and maybe even to a half hour. My sense is that the longer you postpone the binge, the more likely you are to settle for an otherwise innocuous emotional-eating episode, which would be a healthier choice than a binge.

Mindful Emotional Drinking: Water-Drinking Relaxation

awareness &
habit change

So far, we have focused on emotional eating. In addition to eating to cope, people, as we well know, also drink to cope. In the spirit of harm reduction, here's a look at how you can drink to cope without then having to cope with drinking. I invite you to learn to appreciate the relaxing benefits of drinking plain water. Drinking water is a great coping technique: it is simple and can be an effective relaxant. The actual act of drinking prompts you to become more mindful of your breathing to the point of slowing it down enough that you don't choke on the liquid you are about to consume. The preparation of your body for a drink becomes a kind of inadvertent relaxation of breath, which in and of itself is a valid and effective stress-reduction technique. Additionally, the gustatory dynamics of a sip of cold water feel relaxing as well; like a caressing hand, water strokes and soothes the throat and cools the stress-parched mouth. Having a couple of glasses of cold water is a process that, of course, buys you a bit more time to cool off from a stressful situation. Finally, this kind of preloading on water helps you facilitate a quicker onset of fullness and leaves less stomach room to fill with emotional eating, thus helping you prevent emotional overeating.

A Note on Perfection

Have you ever tried to define perfection? Perfection is a state of flawlessness, so immaculate and error free that it cannot be improved upon. Seems beyond reach, doesn't it? Well, it actually isn't. If perfection is a state that cannot be improved upon, then, as strange as it sounds, any moment is perfect in the sense that it has already happened and is too late to improve upon.

Now don't get me wrong: seeing perfection this way is not permission to stop trying. Even though this current moment, as imperfect as it can be, is beyond improvement, the next one still can be better. But before you reject this coping moment as not good enough, allow yourself to accept the imperfect perfection of this moment. And, indeed, if you could cope any more effectively right now, why the hell wouldn't you? In this very moment, you are doing the best you can. If you could already cope with life's stresses without food, of course you would! And right now, you are working on it. Looking at your emotional eating with compassion and making it more mindful will help you eventually attain the pinnacle of food-free coping. But until then, give yourself a pat on the back. It's not as if you haven't been trying.

CHAPTER 5

Meaningful, Not Mouthful

Most eaters, when eating, search for nutrition or comfort or leisure or health. Some search for meaning while eating. Mindfulness and meaningfulness go hand in hand: what is meaningful is typically approached with heightened attention and concentration, and therefore with mindfulness. Explore the activity of eating as a daily opportunity for meaning. Infusing meaningfulness into eating is likely to increase the mindfulness of it as well. Aim to make a paradigm shift from mindless overeating to meaning-centered eating.

Eating as an Expression of Values

Eating, while typically not a conscious part of your worldview, can be made more mindful through a realignment of your eating values with your overall worldview. Vegetarian and vegan traditions are good examples of an attempt to use the activity of eating as a vehicle for the expression of ethics.

Meaningful Eating

awareness To help you infuse meaningfulness into mindless eating, I encourage you to survey your values. Set aside some time to meditate on the following questions: "What is important to me?" "What do I stand for?" "What is life about?" "How do I see my purpose in life?" "What are my goals?" "What do I value?" Write down your answers and brainstorm ways in which your eating can reflect your values.

Eating as Existential Rescue

Believe it or not, the activity of eating takes up about 8 percent of your waking time, which accounts for approximately 1.25 hours per day (Csikszentmihalyi 1998). That's roughly over three years' worth of time just eating (assuming a life expectancy of seventy-five years). That's a lot of time to waste on mindlessness. With this in mind, conscious eating allows you to rescue the moments of your life from the oblivion of mindlessness.

Existential Eating: The Last-Meal Experience

awareness What if this meal were your last? Would you eat it more mindfully? As an exercise, set a date for a pretend last meal. Think about what you'd like for your last meal (both in terms of food and company) and make appropriate arrangements. On the given day, treat yourself to this pseudofarewell meal. Learn from the existential mindfulness of the moment. And, by the way, as you are reading this, how do you know that the meal you are about to eat isn't going to be your last one?

Mindful Eating as Appreciation of Abundance

It has been long observed that some people overeat because they do not want to waste food. Childhood guilt still drives us to clean up our plates. As irrational as it may seem, this guilt trip is based on a reasonable idea of appreciation of abundance. Mindfulness as gratitude for abundance is celebrated on certain holidays, such as Thanksgiving Day, and through various forms of saying grace at each meal. Why not also try to celebrate abundance through mindfulness?

Thankful Eating: Wartime Ration

awareness To appreciate abundance, try to live one day on a daily wartime ration. For example, the daily ration of food in Russia during World War II was as low as 125 grams (about 5 ounces) of bread per day (during the blockade of Leningrad) and a half-inch cube of sugar. But people made it last. They would cut the allowance of bread into several parts and space it throughout the day. They'd often save one or two crouton-shaped pieces of bread for a rainy day or for gestures of goodwill. Sugar was not mixed in with a glass of tea. Instead, a person would take a sip of hot water or tea (if lucky) and briefly suck on a cube of sugar to make it last all day. As you see, mindfulness substituted for the fullness of the stomach. I invite you to research some historical food rations (from wartime or from times of famine) and experiment with having a day in the eating life of an ancestor.

Mindful Eating as an Opportunity for Spirituality

Eating has long been a part of many spiritual traditions. An activity that stitches our days with the regularity of breaths, eating is nothing less than a continuous meditating opportunity, an unexplored reservoir for spiritual recharging that is waiting to be utilized.

Graceful Eating

awareness & habit change One way to capture the meaning of eating is to develop a concise self-address, a sentence that captures the essence of an idea that you are trying to practice. The terminology of this will vary, depending on who you are culturally. So, as the first order of business, you need to decide what you will call this: a sutra, a mantra, grace, a meditation, a prayer, or self-talk. Secondly, you will need to generate a list of statements capturing your intent toward eating. Allow yourself to be creative, daring, metaphorical, and even radical. Express your drive for mindfulness and meaningfulness. Having brainstormed a dozen such statements, select the top three and see if you can combine them into one eating mindfulness sutra/mantra/grace/self-talk. Practice your self-address immediately prior to your eating to instill a new habit of infusing meaningfulness and mindfulness into your eating. Following are a few examples of secular mindful eating self-addresses that you might find meaningful: "I eat to live, not live to eat." "I will eat as if I were eating for the first time in my life; I will eat as if I were eating for the last time in my life." "Food is entertainment enough; I just need to tune in to the action." "Look, smell, taste, pause." "I will be mindful, not mouthful." "Food is medicine: I'll tr-eat but not overdose."

Spiritual Eating Reading Assignment

awareness Here's a reading assignment for you: *Feeding the Body, Nourishing the Soul: Essentials of Eating for Physical, Emotional, and Spiritual Well-Being,* by Deborah Kesten (1997). Kesten's book is a panoramic review of various spiritual applications of eating, spanning the entire spectrum of religious experience. I encourage you to purchase the book and read a chapter a day, just prior to a meal. This is bound to assure at least a couple of weeks' worth of spiritually imbued eating.

Mindful Eating as an Act of Reunification with the Universe

awareness Here's a paragraph from "The Eating Rebel" (Cohn 1996), an article that I came across while writing this book: "Moreover, food is a concentration of the forces of the universe—the sun, the oceans, the wind—going into my body. Those forces, gross and subtle, are unlocked only by chewing food properly. When I remember this, I slow down, becoming an eager locksmith, releasing the energies stored in food. It is easier to practice this idea of unlocking when I don't distract myself during the act of eating."

While the overt suggestion of this quotation is to slow down eating to unlock the energies of the cosmos contained in food, these words also allude to the idea of interconnectedness, with food being a kind of gateway into a never-ending cycle of energy and matter. This is certainly worth a moment of meditation: next time you take a bite or a sip, pause to ponder that in doing so, you are uniting with the universe in a very literal sense. Allow yourself to marvel at the notion that the light that caressed the carrot stick in your hands had to travel for thousands and thousands of years, predating in its origin the very harvest of the carrots you are sampling. Muse over the fact that the apple in your hand is comprised of the molecules and atoms of the same world that was home to generations of your ancestors. Get inspired by the possibility that this fish on your plate might have swum in the same waters as your grandparents on their honeymoon. Take a moment to realize that this food you are about to eat is one of the so-called six degrees of separation that connect you to everything.

Developing Your Own Philosophy of Eating

Let's face it: in trying to manage your overeating, you've been through a lot! You've subjected yourself to the anal-retentive hassle of calorie counting and torturous self-denial through serial dieting. You've gone to boot-camp-style aerobics and spinning classes with nothing more in your stomach than a couple of melon rinds. You've put up with, hopefully, only a probability of anal leakage by subsisting on olestra potato chips. You might have considered or, in fact, undergone one or more weight-loss and cosmetic surgeries, facing the risks of morbidity and mortality. Bottom line: you've been through so much, and there is still so much more to go through. What will guide you on this journey to wellness? Fad diets? I hope not! Perhaps a thought-out philosophy of eating. Don't worry: you don't have to change everything tonight. Nor can you. Making a shift from mindless eating to mindful eating, from eating without a philosophy to eating with a philosophy, is a process, not an event, a process that hopefully has picked up momentum with each awareness-building or habit-modifying exercise you've tried. Now it's time to develop your own philosophy of eating, which is a life-modifying (LM) exercise.

A Life-Modifying Exercise: "My Philosophy of Eating"

life change As I see it, developing your own eating philosophy involves the following three questions:

Question 1: "What purpose will eating hold in my life?"

This is the most important question of the three. Your purpose in eating drives the answers to the other two questions of your philosophy of eating. As you answer this question, avoid "should" thoughts. It is up to you to define the purpose of eating in your life. Consider some possible answers to this question:

Food is fuel: You may decide that eating will only serve the goal of fueling your body and that you will work toward weight loss and maintenance of healthy weight. Makes sense!

Food is therapy: You may decide that eating will fuel your body and satisfy psychological needs. In other words, you will decide that eating will be a form of coping for you. Tr-eat away!

189

Food is socialization: You may decide that eating will serve to bring you close to people. Go ahead, share your appetite!

Food is medicine: You may decide that you will use food as medicine and that you will guide your eating choices by the preventive and healing properties of food. Heal thyself!

Food is longevity: You may decide to use food to help you expand both your health span and lifespan. Live 120 years!

Food is spirituality: You may decide that eating will serve as a regular opportunity for meditation and spirituality. Go ahead and om, not yum!

Food is pleasure: You may proclaim that food is one of life's little pleasures and that you will partake in the hedonism of eating whenever you can. Enjoy!

I am convinced that any of the choices above are compatible with healthy eating, as long as your choice is mindful fueling, mindful emotional eating, mindful socialization through food, mindful self-medication through food, mindful effort to lengthen your days, mindful expression of spirituality through eating, or mindful gustatory hedonism. Each of these eating purposes is compatible with healthy living. Throw away what others say you should do; eating can be anything you want it to be. You don't have to compromise on the quality of your eating life; on the contrary, leverage the quality of your life through mindful eating, whatever the purpose of your eating may be. Finally, can there be more than one purpose to eating? Of course. While some may look at food from a strictly utilitarian standpoint (food equals fuel for body), others may combine eating for health and longevity with eating for spirituality, or for bodily health and emotional self-regulation.

Question 2: "When should I start eating?"

The answer to this question depends on the purpose(s) of your eating. If food is fuel, medicine, or a means to optimize your health span and lifespan, then you should start eating when you experience physiological hunger. If food is self-therapy, then in addition to eating when you are physiologically hungry, it would make sense for you to eat when you are hungry for emotional well-being, as long as you do it with mindfulness. If food is socialization, then give yourself the permission to mingle eating with mingling, guiltlessly, as long as you do it with a good degree of mindfulness. If food is a source of hedonistic pleasure, once again allow yourself to enjoy it guilt free, even if you are not hungry, as long as you do so in moderation and with mindfulness.

Question 3: "When should I stop eating?"

Once again, the answer to this question is driven by the purpose(s) of your eating. If food is fuel, medicine, or a means of assuring your health span and lifespan, then you should stop eating whenever you experience the relief of hunger and no later than the onset of pleasant fullness. If food is a source of pleasure, then, by definition, it would make sense to stop no later than the onset of pleasant fullness. If food is self-therapy, then whenever you eat to cope, it would make sense to stop as soon as you have attained a desired emotional state. If food is a vehicle for socializing, stop when you are pleasantly full. While sitting down to eat with somebody is, indeed, key to socializing through eating, you are unlikely to jeopardize your social connection by pushing away from the table whenever you feel physiologically ready.

What Are the Implications of Your Eating Philosophy?

As this book draws to a close, it is time for you to tie together the strings of meaning and mindfulness into a life-modifying knot. Allow yourself a pensive moment to conclude your searching with a summary of your eating philosophy and its implications. Here are a few examples to help you start this roundup of ideas. Depending on the purpose(s) of eating in your life, your eating philosophy might sound as follows:

Food as fuel, socialization, and a means of emotional self-help: "I will use food primarily to maintain healthy weight and occasionally as a form of coping with emotional distress.

Therefore, I will eat when I am physiologically hungry as a rule, with the occasional exception of eating out, even if I do not feel true physiological hunger, for the purpose of socializing or when I feel upset. I will aim to stop eating when I reach pleasant fullness or when I have attained the desired emotional relief."

Food as pleasure only: "I will use food as a source of pleasure. I like to eat and I am not ashamed of it. I am choosing to eat for fun. I will also strive to offset any health hazards of using food for fun by learning to enjoy healthy foods with disease-preventive properties. I will also offset any health hazards of using food for fun by preventing overeating. To this aim, I will eat what I want but only when I am physiologically hungry, and I will stop eating when I am pleasantly full. I realize that eating hedonistically (and I use this term without judgment) might not help me lose weight. Therefore, I recognize the need to offset my reliance on food for pleasure with adequate exercise."

Food as medicine and a means to longevity: "I will use food as both reactive and preventive medicine and as a way to extend the longevity of my health span and lifespan. Therefore, I choose to eat only when I am physiologically hungry and stop eating when I feel I have relieved my physiological hunger and/or have eaten a sufficient dosage of food with the medicinal and nutritive properties I am trying to benefit from."

Food as fuel for body and mind/soul: "I will use eating as an opportunity, in the words of Deborah Kesten, to both 'feed the body' and to 'nourish the soul.' Therefore, I will approach my meals with mindfulness, appreciating each meal as a solitary or social spiritual opportunity or an opportunity for meaning. I will remain mindful throughout my meals and end them on a note of moderation and balance, avoiding unpleasant fullness whenever I can. I will recognize meals as daily opportunities for existential and/or spiritual realignment and practice meaningful, not mouthful, eating. At times, when it is necessary, after I've made an adequate attempt to cope with life's stressors without food, I will, with moderation, eat to cope, remembering not to overdose on chicken soup for the soul or its secular equivalent, egg drop soup for the mind."

I Wish You Well!

You, the reader, and I, the author of these tentative ideas, begin to part ways. From here, you are on your own. But remember that you now have the power of mindfulness and the guidance of your eating philosophy.

References

Cheney, D. 2006. *Tasting Club: Gathering Together to Share and Savor Your Favorite Tastes*. New York: DK Publishing.

Cohn, A. 1996. The eating rebel. Magic Stream. http://magic stream.org/ari.htm.

Craighead, L. W. 2006. *Appetite Awareness Training*. Oakland, CA: New Harbinger Publications.

Crawford, D. C., and E. Sounder. 1995. Smell disorders = danger. *RN* 58 (11):40–4.

Csikszentmihalyi, M. 1998. *Finding Flow: The Psychology of Engagement with Everyday Life*. New York: Basic Books.

Dennett, D. C. 1992. *Consciousness Explained*. Boston: Back Bay Books.

Duffy, V. B., J. R. Backstrand, and A. M. Ferris. 1995. Olfactory dysfunction and related nutritional risk in free-living elderly women. *Journal of the American Dietetic Association* 95 (8): 879–85.

Fletcher, J. 2000. The fifth taste: Elusive taste dimension can mean the difference between balance and blah. *San Francisco Chronicle,* July 5, fd-1.

Fuhrman, J. 2003. *Eat to Live*. New York: Little, Brown, and Company.

Gladwell, M. 2007. *Blink: The Power of Thinking Without Thinking*. Boston: Back Bay Books.

Green, B. G., M. Alvarez-Reeves, and P. George. 2005. Chemesthesis and taste: Evidence of independent processing of sensation intensity. *Physiology and Behavior* 86 (4):526–37.

Hetherington, M. M., and B. J. Rolls. 1996. Sensory-specific satiety: Theoretical framework and characteristics. In *Why We Eat What We Eat: The Psychology of Eating,* ed. by E. D. Capaldi. Washington, DC: American Psychological Association.

Hirsch, A. R. 1998. *Scentsational Weight Loss: At Last, a New, Easy, Natural Way to Control Your Appetite.* New York: Fireside Books.

Holt, S. H., J. C. Miller, P. Petocz, and E. Farmakalidis. 1995. A satiety index of common foods. *European Journal of Clinical Nutrition* 49 (9):675–90.

Kesten, D. 1997. *Feeding the Body, Nourishing the Soul: Essentials of Eating for Physical, Emotional, and Spiritual Well-Being.* Berkeley, CA: Conari Press.

Krasner, J. 2006. This dieting aid smells like victory to start-up. *The Boston Globe,* December 7, D1.

Marlatt, G. A. 2002a. Buddhist philosophy and the treatment of addictive behavior. *Cognitive and Behavioral Practice* 9: 44–50.

———. 2002b. *Harm Reduction: Pragmatic Strategies for Managing High-Risk Behaviors.* New York: The Guilford Press.

Raynor, H. A., and L. H. Epstein. 2001. Dietary variety, energy regulation, and obesity. *Psychological Bulletin* 127 (3):325–41.

Roth, G., and A. Lamott. 1999. *When You Eat at the Refrigerator, Pull Up a Chair.* New York: Hyperion Books.

Tribole, E., and E. Resch. 1996. *Intuitive Eating: A Recovery Book for the Chronic Dieter: Rediscover the Pleasure of Eating and Rebuild Your Body Image.* New York: St. Martin's Press.

Uijtdehaage, S. H., R. M. Stern, and K. L. Koch. 1992. Effects of eating on vection-induced motion sickness, cardiac vagal tone, and gastric myoelectrical activity. *Psychophysiology* 29 (2):193–201.

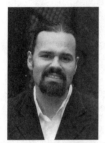

Photo by John Colombo
www.johncolombo.com

Pavel G. Somov. Ph.D., is a clinical psychologist in private practice in Pittsburgh, PA. The mindful-eating program presented in this book uses techniques and tools he developed for his clients. He has successfully used similar mindfulness-based interventions with substance abusers in recovery. Somov emigrated from Russia at the age of twenty-one and became a US citizen in 1996. He received his Ph.D. in counseling psychology from the State University of New York at Buffalo in 2000.

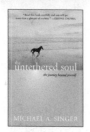
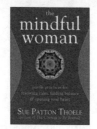
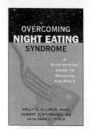
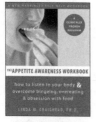
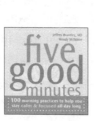
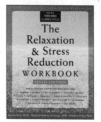
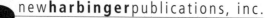